Candida
Directory

Candida Directory

Helen Gustafson
& Maureen O'Shea

With recipes by
Jennifer Ali ∘ Anni Amberger-Warren
Sharon Cadwallader ∘ Dorothy Calimeris ∘ Julia Child
Chandra Cho ∘ Marion Cunningham ∘ Narsai David ∘ Anne Fox
Jill Gustafson ∘ Tatiana Krabbe ∘ Dayna Macy
Jackie Mallorca ∘ Rosemary Manell ∘ Wolfgang Puck
Charles Shere ∘ Peggy Smith ∘ Alice Waters

CELESTIAL ARTS
Berkeley, California

Winter Vegetable Cobbler from *The Fanny Farmer Cookbook, 13th revised edition*
by Marion Cunningham. Copyright © 1990 by Marion Cunningham. Reprinted
by permission of Alfred A. Knopf, Inc.

Poached Fish Steaks with Lemon Butter Sauce, Braised Celery, Celery Rave, and
Garlic Mashed Potatoes from *From Julia Child's Kitchen* by Julia Child. Copyright
© 1975 by Julia Child. Reprinted by permission of Alfred A. Knopf, Inc.

Bay Scallops with Sautéed Apples from *The Wolfgang Puck Cookbook* by Wolfgang
Puck. Copyright © 1986 by Wolfgang Puck. Reprinted by permission of Random
House, Inc.

Tofu Steaks from *The Reluctant Cook* by Helen Gustafson. Copyright © 1990 by
Helen Gustafson. Reprinted by permission of Celestial Arts Publishing, Inc.

Cover design by Fifth Street Design
Text design and typography by FORM FOLLOWS FUNCTION
First Printing 1994

Library of Congress Cataloging in Publication Data

Gustafson, Helen.
The candida directory : the comprehensive guide to yeast-free living / by
Helen Gustafson & Maureen O'Shea.
                           p.   cm.
Includes bibliographical references and index.
        ISBN-13: 978-0-89087-714-2
        ISBN-10: 0-89087-714-9
1. Candidiasis—Diet therapy.   2. Candidiasis—Directories.   I. O'Shea,
Maureen.   II. Title.
RC123.C3G87 1994
818.9'89—dc20   93-50920
                                    CIP

12   13 / 10   09   08

Acknowledgments

THIS BOOK GREW out of a vigorous search for recipes to use in controlling yeast. Helen had been diagnosed with Candida albicans a month before, and Maureen, a nutritional consultant, had been recommended to her as someone who could help with the diet. After going through a bewildering pile of "pretty good books," we simultaneously burst out, "Someday I'm going to write a book about this!" and an instant partnership was formed.

Helen would like to thank the following:

Sandra Wooten, Rosen worker and miracle worker; Mijo Horwich for her hands-on-care and daily encouragement; Dr. Carol Jessop who diagnosed my condition; Dr. Hilda Burton for truthfulness and support; and Daide Donnelly for congratulating me on being obsessive.

Maureen would like to thank the following:

Dr. William Lockyer, one of the few physicians who meets the Latin definition of doctor: *one who teaches;* Dr. Linda Berry who so graciously shared her knowledge over of the years; Dr. Daniel Donner for his healing care; the memory of Dr. Phyllis L. Saifer, whose years of work and devotion helped so many find their paths to wellness; my husband, Lynn and daughter, Christina, for hanging in with me the whole way; all my dear friends and colleagues who cheered me on; and all the clients who have taught me so much over the years.

Helen and Maureen would both like to thank:

Sal Glynn for his magnificent editorial genius; Claire O'Shea for her legal guidance; Clair Gustafson for advice and support; Anne Fox for her complete and thorough devotion to our book as recipe editor; and most of all Dr. Miki Shima for his healing spirit, his sensitve perceptions, and inexhaustible knowledge. We'd also like to thank our recipe contributors: Jennifer Ali, Anni Amberger-Warren, Sharon Cadwallader, Dorothy Calimeris, Julia Child, Chandra Cho, Marion Cunningham, Narsai David, Anne Fox, Jill Gustafson, Tatiana Krabbe, Dayna Macy, Jackie Mallorca, Rosemary Manell, Wolfgang Puck, Charles Shere, Peggy Smith, and Alice Waters.

Helen's Dedication
For Pat MacDonald, superb medical technician who, upon commiserating with me on my diagnosis, said, "Well, there's your next book."

Maureen's Dedication
To my dear friend Judith Tsagris, who taught me the importance of consciousness and whose loving friendship I've cherished over the years.

Table of Contents

Introduction

CANDIDA ALBICANS, COMMONLY known as yeast, a normal component of the body, ordinarily lives in harmony with acidophilus, the "good bacteria," that aids digestion and elimination. But antibiotics, hormones, birth control pills, and steroids can suppress acidophilus, allowing yeast to grow unchecked. This yeast reacts just as does the yeast used in baking. When warm water and sugar are added to commercial yeast, it bubbles up so rapidly it almost seems to explode. Yeast acts in much the same way in your body if the internal flora is unbalanced.

Unfortunately, the typical all-American diet works against a natural balance of yeast and acidophilus. Over-processed foods, refined carbohydrates, alcoholic beverages and sugar, sugar, sugar (in everything imaginable, including soups) are foods which encourage yeast growth, making the body a paradise for Candida. Tucked away in a dark, warm, protected place and regularly fed what it loves, why should the yeast agree to leave such a "land of plenty?"

Indeed, once yeast has colonized the body it becomes quite a task to drive it out. The original Candida diet, designed to stunt yeast, eliminated all sweeteners, fruit (and fruit juices), dried or fermented foods, and foods that attract mold. Carbohydrates were ruled out completely. Meat and vegetables, prepared in the blandest way, were left. Physicians soon discovered that patients who had been placed on this radical diet were staggering around weak and dispirited. As a result, some complex carbohydrates have been allowed in amounts that depend on the patient's tolerance.

Maureen, who has been working with Candida patients for ten years, developed a program for Helen that allowed her not only manageable amounts of complex carbohydrates but also safe levels of other "taboo" foods. Our effort in this book has been to offer guidelines for a diet you can live with—in the true sense of the phrase. We will help you cleanse and rebalance your system, making Candida a problem that you can solve.

Helen's yeast problem was more than an intense craving for ice cream, breads, and sweet rolls. She had other classic reactions to yeast grown beyond its bounds: mysterious fatigue, sore throats, swollen glands, aching joints, and unsteady balance—all with no fever. These symptoms suggested that an overgrowth of yeast, or Candida, had produced toxins which were triggering her immune system to react.

The unsteady balance and awkwardness which Helen experienced is in keeping with a famous Candida case which showed there's more than one way to get tipsy.

A gentleman from Phoenix, Charles M. Swaart, treated himself to a large Italian meal that included an antipasto plate, pasta with tomato sauce, mushrooms, cheese, and French bread. He followed dinner with a luxuriously sweet dessert. Throughout the meal Charles had only water to drink, but he reeled out of the restaurant, causing the police to stop him on his way home. As they expected, Charles' blood showed a high level of alcohol. He protested that he had imbibed nothing alcoholic, a fact corroborated by the restaurant owner. Charles took his case to court and won. Why then, the high level of alcohol? Dr. Kazuo Iwata, a professor of microbiology at the University of Tokyo School of Medicine, having seen many similar cases of "drunkenness disease" in Japan, contacted Charles and his current physician, Dr. Frances Sierakowski.

The two doctors discovered that Charles' level of Candida was already out of balance and that the intense meal of refined carbohydrates dramatically increased it. The multiplying yeast quickly produced their natural waste product, alcohol, and it was recorded in the blood test.

If you've been diagnosed with Candida, or have been stumbling around looking for a diet that will bring your system into balance, start with the Symptom Chart (page 6). It comes from Maureen's years of work with the late Phyllis Saifer, M. D., a well-recognized environmental allergist. Instead of having to rely on your memory (which can be so unreliable, especially when you're sick), match your present state of mind and body with the symptoms listed on the chart. Use this chart throughout the three-stage program to monitor your progress. Knowing what step you're on enables you to plan the next one.

To get well quickly and efficiently, make a list of grocery items you might want and then check it against the Food Directory (page 153). In a matter of seconds you can see which foods can be eaten and which needs to be handled with care or included in the later stages of your diet. Pears, for instance, are taboo at the beginning of the diet but fine later in the program.

The recipes show Helen's devotion to eating well no matter what. From her friends in the world of food, she's gathered recipes of famous chefs throughout the country. In the appendices, you'll also be able to find sources for supplements, vitamins and special foods no matter where you live, saving the lengthy telephone search that many (including the authors) have endured. Finally, you'll find tips on how to view your condition and to manage it successfully as you go.

One bit of wisdom: this diet is not forever. It will lead you to wellness, and from there you eat to stay in balance. Keep in mind that Candida is a problem you can control. Start each day with a positive, heartfelt desire to eliminate excess yeast—but don't think of "starving" it. Psychologically you may feel that you are starving. Not true! In fact you will thrive as the yeast shrinks back to normal levels, brought under control by a diet which is both tasty and healthful. Enjoy looking forward to meals, and to yourself looking clear-eyed (even glamorous) and feeling healthy.

Fill out the Symptom Chart to begin mapping your path to Stage II. Once you get into the rhythm of moving through the stages, your journey back to health will be a pleasant ride. Bon voyage and bon appétit!

How to Use This Book

1. Copies of Stage I, the Eat/Avoid List, and the Symptom Chart should be made out immediately. Consult the Food Directory for a quick and convenient reference guide. Use Candida Antifungal Preparations (page 53) along with the Mail Order Food Sources (page 189) as desired.

2. Look at the recipe section and figure out a meal plan for the week ahead (see Suggested Meal Plan for Stage I on page 74).

3. Take acidophilus daily (page 57) and a good multiple vitamin/mineral (page 59). If you are not under someone's care, consider taking some sort of antifungal preparation (page 55) like grapefruit seed extract or caprillyic acid to help eliminate the Candida. See page 52 on how to eliminate "die-off" when first starting to kill the yeast.

4. Proceed with Stage I for three weeks and then fill out the Symptom Chart once more. Follow the Calculations to decide your progress from thereon. If you've successfully completed Stage I, then simply repeat the above three steps in Stage II.

   If you must remain on Stage I, continue another three weeks and try again. Keep repeating this pattern until you are able to proceed to Stage II.

5. When you have reached Stage III, along with the other obvious prizes (cheese, bread, mushrooms, and others), you'll be able to eat out again with moderate restrictions.

6. If you can now eat everything that's listed on Stage III, with your doctor's blessing, you can consider yourself as having completed the stages of the journey.

Section One

About Candida Albicans
and the Candida Diet

Do You Have Candida Albicans?

☐ Do you feel tired most of the time?

☐ Do you suffer from intestinal gas, abdominal bloating, or discomfort?

☐ Do you crave sugar, breads, or beer and other alcoholic beverages?

☐ Are you bothered by constipation, diarrhea, or alternating constipation and diarrhea?

☐ Do you suffer from mood swings or depression?

☐ Are you often irritable, easily angered, anxious, or nervous?

☐ Do you have trouble thinking clearly, suffer occasional memory losses, or have difficulty concentrating?

☐ Are you ever dizzy or light-headed?

☐ Do your muscles ache or stiffen with normal activity?

☐ Have you had experienced weight gain without change in diet?

☐ Are you bothered by itching or burning of the vagina or prostate, or loss of sexual desire?

☐ Have you ever taken antibiotics?

☐ Are you currently using or have you ever used birth control pills?

☐ Have you ever taken steroid drugs, such as cortisone?

Rate your answers with this chart:

Number of yes answers	Probability of a yeast infection
11 or more	very high
7 to 10	high
5 to 6	moderate
4 or less	low

Chapter One

🌿

What Are Your Symptoms?

I N 1988, HELEN had a morning conference with a therapist friend who had undergone a long period of immune system dysfunction. Before their meeting Helen had once again hauled out all her papers, notes, flyers, newsletters and books on Candida—each more confusing and full of useless "inspirational" stories than the last. As they spoke, Helen was feeling tense and hungry after her usual unsatisfying breakfast of scrambled eggs, hot water, and rye crackers.

Her friend, usually kind and even-tempered, suddenly confounded her with what seemed a particularly cruel statement: "Hmm—you seem rather obsessive." Helen's reserve broke, and she shot back, "Yes, of course, I am. I want to get well!" The unspoken "you idiot" was in her tone. The friend smiled, sat back in her chair and said, "Good. You have to be obsessive if you're going to get better." How the air cleared! Doubts about fussing with herself and her family to get rid of this problem faded. She felt vindicated, correct, and smart.

They began to review everything they could about Helen's life. There were her eating and energy patterns, supplements, how much water and what kind she drank, exercise and rest (mostly rest!), health history, emotional state, home environment, and family history. Helen's friend told her about the long trial-and-error period she herself had slogged through. It took over two years for her to realize that fish at dinner caused her friend to ache and be depressed the next day. Two years! "There are so many factors to consider," she said. "It takes a long time to sift and sort them all out." If only she had a symptom chart!

The Symptom Chart which follows will help you make discoveries quickly and speed you on the way to health.

Ten years of counseling experience with patients enabled Maureen to develop this chart, and it acts as a guide to help you judge your progress. As you use the Symptom Chart, you will know when to progress through the stages of the diet. You'll find an example of how to fill out the chart on page 7 and an interpretation in the Calculations on page 6. We hope the Calculations will be fairly simple for you. The values used there are merely guidelines, not absolute figures.

Even with a partial use of the chart, you'll be doing something about your condition, immediately taking some control over your life, and improving your sense of well-being. But to really know when to proceed through the stages of the diet, you need to work with this chart. That may mean enlisting someone to help you with this task like Helen did with her friend. For more advice on how to ask someone for help, see page 66.

What is Candida Albicans?

Candida albicans lives in our bodies from the moment we are born. Under normal conditions, your body can control the amount of yeast you have. Under certain circumstances, such as a weakened constitution, allergies, use of antibiotics, steroids and hormones, yeast overgrowth may occur. When such an overgrowth occurs, things get out of control. This excessive amount of Candida in your body can then set up a variety of physiological conditions or symptoms.

Your immune system produces antibodies to fight against the yeast cells, which are perceived as intruders. If you have other immune problems, such as allergies or viruses, the antibodies of the immune system become overworked, sensitivities to pollens, foods, tobacco smoke, perfumes, or chemicals can increase. Though yeast lives mostly in the mucous membranes of the mouth, sinus, stomach, vaginal cavity or intestines, it can also affect joints and muscles in the form of aches and stiffness, as well as the skin, in the way of rashes or athlete's foot.

Dead yeast cells are equally harmful: they produce toxins that your body reacts to in different ways. The liver may function poorly. Cells may fail to communicate with each other. You may experience memory loss and/or confusion.

Because your entire body can be affected by Candida's overgrowth, all symptoms must be taken into consideration. On the following page you'll find the Symptom Chart which you will use to list your symptoms in detail. Please note that during the course of treatment, **some symptoms may not improve because they are not related to yeast. If such problems persist, make sure to discuss other possible causes with your doctor.** You may also feel worse when starting the diet if you are simultaneously taking some anti-fungal medication or preparation. As yeast cells die, they produce toxic substances which can cause headaches, joint pain, nausea, and tiredness. Generally, the period of "die-off" caused by anti-fungal treatments lasts anywhere from four days to thirty days, depending on how your treatment is increased during this period. (For more information about how anti-fungal treatments can affect you, see chapter three, Candida Antifungal Preparations and How They Work on page 51.)

Use the Symptom Chart every three weeks to check your progress and determine when you should move on to the the next stages of the diet. The Calculations will help you figure out when to proceed.

Calculations

1. Three weeks after you've started using the Symptom Chart, count up the checked symptoms recorded on the date you started.

2. Count the better and cleared symptoms you recorded three weeks after the starting date.

3. Using the example below, determine your percentage of improvement.

EXAMPLE:

Date Started: 8/3/94
A. Total symptoms as of 8/3 = 30
B. Total better and cleared symptoms as of 8/24 = 10
C. To get the percentage of improvement divide B by A and multiply that number by 100. 10 ÷ 30 = .33 x 100 = 33% improvement

4. Depending upon your percentage of improvement, do one of the following:
   a. If you have less than fifty percent improvement, stay on Stage I for three more weeks.
   b. If you have fifty percent or more improvement, go on to Stage II of the diet.

5. If you've been on Stage II long enough to have added all of the foods suggested and you are fifty percent improved, then go on to Stage III.

6. Starting Stage III can be stressful if you are very mold-sensitive. Remember to avoid mold-family foods (cheeses, mushrooms, bakers yeast, and brewer's yeast) during mold season (marked by rainy, foggy, or humid weather).

Symptom Chart

Make several copies of the following blank forms to work on during the diet. Use the left-hand column to check your symptoms from the date started. Every three weeks check your progress, comparing the current date with the last date. Use the symbols in the legend to evaluate your symptoms. The Calculations will help you see your progress every three weeks. The following example will show you how to proceed:

Sample Symptom Chart

Legend: **W=Worse   S=Same   B=Better   G=Gone**

Date started	Symptom	Date	Date	Date	Date	Date
8/3	**Nerves and feelings**	*8/24*	*9/14*	*10/5*	*10/26*	*11/6*
	Anxiety					
	Apathy					
✔	Confusion	W	B	B	B	G
	Depression					
	Dizziness					
	Fainting					
✔	Fatigue	S	B	B	G	G
	Feelings of rage					
✔	Forgetfulness	W	W	S	B	G
	Hallucinations					
✔	Headache	W	S	B	G	G
	Hyperactivity					
	Insomnia/nightmares					
	Irritability					
	Learning disorders					
	Migraine					

Notice how headache became worse after starting, then remained the same for the next three week period. By 10/15 headache got better, and by 10/26 finally cleared and remained that way on 11/16.

Symptom Chart

Date started	Symptom	Date	Date	Date	Date	Date
	Nerves and feelings					
	Anxiety					
	Apathy					
	Confusion					
	Depression					
	Dizziness					
	Fainting					
	Fatigue					
	Feelings of rage					
	Forgetfulness					
	Hallucinations					
	Headache					
	Hyperactivity					
	Insomnia/nightmares					
	Irritability					
	Learning disorders					
	Migraine					
	Mood swings					
	Numbness and tingling					
	Poor concentration					
	Seizures					

Symptom Chart

Date started	Date	Date	Date	Date	Date
Sleepiness					
Spacey feelings					
Other					
Skin					
Acne					
Athlete's foot					
Body fungus					
Dandruff					
Dryness/oiliness					
Flushing					
Itching					
Pallor					
Rash (hives/eczema/other)					
Sores/infections					
Other					
Eyes and vision					
Blurring					
Burn					
Circles under eyes					
Itching					
Pain					
Puffy eyes					
Red eyes					

Symptom Chart

Date started		Date	Date	Date	Date	Date
	Sensitive to light					
	Spots/floaters					
	Tearing					
	Other					
	Ears					
	Earache					
	Extreme sensitivity to sound					
	Full/blocked/pressure					
	Itching					
	Ringing in ears					
	Other					
	Nasal					
	Itchy nose					
	Nosebleeds					
	Post-nasal drip					
	Runny nose					
	Sinus discomfort/face pain					
	Sneezing fits					
	Stuffy nose					
	Other					
	Throat, mouth, and gums					
	Bad metallic taste/bad breath					
	Canker sores					

Symptom Chart

Date started	Date	Date	Date	Date	Date
Choking					
Coated tongue					
Difficulty in swallowing					
Dry lips					
Hoarse voice					
Increased salivation					
Itching					
Mucus					
Sensitive teeth					
Soreness					
Swolleness					
Tightness in throat					
Other					
Lymph system					
Swollen, tender glands					
Blood vessels					
Chilly feeling					
Cold hands and feet					
Generalized swelling					
Low/high blood pressure					
Low body temperature					
Puffy face					
Spontaneous bruising					

Symptom Chart

Date started	Date	Date	Date	Date	Date
Sweating					
Other					
Heart and lungs					
Chest pain					
Coughing					
Difficulty in breathing					
Pounding pulse					
Rapid breathing					
Rapid or irregular pulse					
Shortness of breath					
Tightness in chest					
Wheezing					
Other					
Gastro/intestinal					
Belching					
Burning sensation					
Constipation					
Cramps					
Diarrhea					
Fullness/bloating					
Gas					
Hunger/thirst					
Nausea					

Symptom Chart

Date started	Date	Date	Date	Date	Date
Pain					
Rectal itch					
Rumbling					
Stomach ache					
Soiling					
Vomiting					
Other					
Weight problem					
Easy gain					
Easy loss					
Fluid retention					
Food aversions					
Food cravings					
Night eating					
Need to gain					
Need to lose					
Other					
Genito/urinary					
Bed wetting					
Breast swelling					
Frequent urination					
Impotence					
Loss of libido					

Symptom Chart

Date started	Date	Date	Date	Date	Date
Menstrual irregularities					
Painful urination					
Urgency to urinate					
Vaginal discharge					
Yeast infections					
Other					
Muscles					
Aching/pain: neck, back, legs					
Shakiness: neck, back, legs					
Weakness: neck, back, legs					
Other					
Joints					
Aches					
Red/warm					
Swelling					
Other					

Chapter Two

❦

The Three Stages
of the Candida Diet

OST CANDIDA DIETS require staying on some type of food program until you are well. The original program was just meat and vegetables, with no carbohydrates (grains and beans) or sweetener of any kind. The reduced carbohydrates coupled with large amounts of meat were a problem for many, particularly vegetarians. Fermented and dried foods (vinegar and herbs) were eliminated along with mold foods (cheeses, mushrooms, and yeasted breads) so that the immune system could focus on the eliminating the Candida. All of these eliminated foods were left out of the diet until it was over.

Our Candida diet is designed to answer different needs. In Stage I you start eating foods to discourage yeast's growth and strengthen your immune system, as in the original diet. But there will be no carbohydrate restrictions in your selection of complex carbohydrates *unless,* you suffer from carbohydrate intolerance.

Carbohydrate Intolerance

Carbohydrate intolerance refers to someone who can't eat a lot of carbohydrate. Generally speaking, people who fall under this category know who they are by their reactions to eating foods such as potatoes, artichokes, brown rice, beans, fruits, and refined grains.

Most carbohydrate intolerant types are left only meat and vegetables as non-reactive foods.

If you think or suspect that you might be carbohydrate intolerant, limit the following foods in the first part of Stage I:

all listed whole grains (rice, whole wheat, corn, and rye)

all listed legumes (soybeans, beans, lentils, and peas)

all listed nuts

artichoke, potato (both white and sweet), yam, parsnip, shallot, leek, garlic, squash, pumpkin, and rutabaga

Cooking vegetables increases their carbohydrate value, so eating raw vegetables is the best choice. By using some form of antifungal medication you'll progress to a level where you will not have to restrict these foods. Once this happens you can continue with the rest of the stages of the diet as indicated.

Carbohydrate Value of Fruit

When first selecting a piece of fruit from the list, pick a choice that is relatively low in carbohydrates. For instance, you may wish to start with strawberries, apricots, tangerines, or peaches. Try to keep your selection between ten and twenty carbohydrate points a day when first adding fruit. Each selection is considered one serving of fruit. Begin with one serving and progress to two servings when you are further along in the program. As you progress you may select items from the twenty to thirty gram range. A chart follows on page 18.

Mold Intolerance and Allergies

If you've been tested and know you're sensitive to environmental mold or if you are intolerant to various molds, do not add mold family foods during mold season. Anyone with a mold problem should (regardless of the season) always peel cucumber and potato skins, and watch out for moldy onion skins and berries. Mold season occurs during winter or any time it is rainy, foggy, or overcast. Increased humidity (above fifty percent) during these weather conditions allows mold spores to come out and be present in the air. During lower humidity (less than fifty percent) the mold spores remain dormant and will not present a problem. Choose days with low humidity to try a mold family food if you are mold sensitive. If you still react to mold family foods on days of low humidity, refrain from eating more until you are finished with diet.

If you are not sensitive to environmental mold or are not mold intolerant, just pay attention to your symptoms when adding other foods. Try the food and if you react, wait four days and try again. If you react again, wait two weeks and try again.

If you aren't sure you are sensitive to environmental mold and you notice a reaction from eating a mold family food, stop eating the food, wait for four days and try it again. If you are still reacting and the humidity is above fifty percent, wait for better weather and try again. If after observing the weather you still react, wait for two weeks and try again.

Mold foods are eliminated from the diet because they can add stress to the immune system. When the immune system no longer has to respond to both Candida and the moldy foods, it becomes less reactive, focusing more on the elimination of Candida. If you have a compromised immune system (AIDS, cancer, or severe Chronic Fatigue Syndrome), consider keeping mold family foods out of your diet to maximize your recovery.

Some Healthy Eating Tips about Protein

The recommended daily amount of protein for adult males is about fifty-six grams and forty-four grams for adult females. Most Americans eat twice these amounts in one day. The daily diet used to revolve around large amounts of animal protein (chicken, beef, and pork) and dairy (milk and milk products), with very little amounts of grains (wheat, corn, oats, and rye) and legumes (soybeans, beans, lentils, and peas).

Carbohydrate Value of Fruit

Name	Carbohydrates	Quantity
Apple, unpeeled	21.5	1 apple, medium
Apricot	11.8	3 apricots
Avocado		
California	6.0	½ avocado
Florida	14.0	½ avocado
Banana	27.0	1 banana
Blackberry	18.4	1 cup
Blueberry	20.5	1 cup
Cherries, sour	18.9	1 cup
Figs, raw	28.5	3 figs
Grapefruit	30.21	½ grapefruit, medium
Lemon		
peeled	5.5	1 lemon
juice	10.5	1 cup
Orange, peeled	15.4	1 orange
Papaya	13.7	1 cup
Peach	9.7	1 peach, medium
Pear		
Bartlett	25.10	1 pear
Bosc	21.3	1 pear
Persimmon		
Hochiya	19.7	1 persimmon
Fuyu	33.5	1 persimmon
Pineapple, diced	19.2	1 cup
Plum		
Japanese	8.6	1 plum
Prune type	6.0	1 plum
Raspberries, red	16.7	1 cup raspberries
Strawberries, capped	10.5	1 cup strawberries
Tangerines	9.4	1 tangerine

Today's health advocates recommend less or no meat, with lots of grains, legumes, and vegetables. The daily recommended dietary plan of the nineties calls for six to eleven servings of grains, four to six servings of vegetables and beans, two to three servings of low or nonfat dairy choices, and one to two servings of animal protein. Eating this way can greatly enhance your health and longevity. If you are an already a practicing vegetarian or have been wanting to eat less animal protein here are some basic tips to consider:

The following combinations can be eaten up to six hours apart. Refer to the Eat/Avoid charts to find all of the members of the grains, legumes, and nuts and seeds food groups:

> A grain and a legume equals a complete protein.
>
> A grain and a legume and nuts or seeds equals a complete protein.
>
> Nuts or seeds and a legume equals a complete protein.
>
> Nuts or seeds and a grain doesn't equal a complete protein.

Here are some other high quality protein combinations:

> Kale, collard greens, mustard greens, Swiss chard, beet greens, winter squash, sweet potato, or yam with any legume.
>
> Fresh lima beans, peas, Brussels sprouts, collard greens, spinach, broccoli, asparagus, okra, snap green beans or cauliflower with any grain, especially corn.
>
> Spinach, mustard green, broccoli, collard greens, corn, okra, or soybean with potatoes.

Sometimes other health conditions (AIDS, Chronic Fatigue Syndrome, or cancer) can affect meat-eaters and vegetarians in different ways. Your health advocate (doctor, acupuncturist, chiropractor, or nutritionist) might suggest changing your existing meal plan for different reasons. A long-term vegetarian with AIDS might be told to eat an animal protein like fish, two or three times a week. A meat eater with cancer may be asked to focus on a vegetarian meal plan. Someone who is allergic to wheat or is carbohydrate intolerant (unable to eat grains, legumes and starchy vegetables) will need to eat more animal protein. It becomes very difficult to recommend one general way of eating with so many different individual circumstances to consider. Remember that general recommendations are for a broad spectrum of people.

As your journey through the three stages progresses, you can gradually increase your food choices to continuously improve your overall nutrition. By Stage II fruits, dried/fermented foods, refined grains, and milk are possible selections. By the completion of Stage III all moldy foods, walnuts, and melons are included. Such foods are not inherently detrimental to your system. Once you have restored your body's acidophilus-yeast balance, a whole host of food choices are again possible.

Throughout the entire diet all sweeteners, alcoholic beverages, and drinks with caffeine are excluded. Not only do these items lack nutritional value, they are also major players in the overgrowth of yeast.

In the Food Directory you'll find a large assortment of food items, some of which may seem exotic or out of the ordinary to you. Yet the recipes themselves are made with basic ingredients for the everyday grocery store shopper. This may at first appear to be a contradiction. However, if you can purchase quinoa, or other foods of nutritional value that are listed, we encourage you to eat them along with the recipes. A balanced, diversified diet of whole foods (grains, legumes, meats, and vegetables) will speed you along the road to recovery.

We hope that you will find your journey through this diet to be a pleasant and rewarding experience.

Stage One Instructions

1. If you have not already done so, fill out the Symptom Chart on page 6 before you begin the diet.

2. Create a daily meal plan from any of the foods listed in Stage I. See the Meal Plan on page 74 for some suggestions. Go shopping and cook ahead.

3. Plan to have enough food in your kitchen for five days so that you can easily fix breakfast, lunch, and dinner. If you're not home for a meal, take it with you. Be sure you have plenty of good snacks (carrot sticks, almonds, raw cauliflower, and plain yogurt). See Mavericks on page 95 for some tasty snacks.

4. Try to eat a variety of different vegetables and grains. You may notice unfamiliar foods listed in Stage I and in the Food List. Be daring and try something new! Check the Mail Order Food Sources on page 189 to help you find some of these exotic foods. Also try shopping at health food stores or ethnic markets (Latin American, Japanese, or Chinese).

5. Follow Stage I for three weeks and then fill out the Symptom Chart again to see if you've improved. If the calculations for the Symptom Chart indicate that you can go on, follow the instructions on page 29 for Stage II. If you have not improved at least fifty percent, continue on Stage I for another three weeks and repeat filling out the Symptom Chart. Stay on Stage I until your calculations from the Symptom Chart indicate that you can go on to Stage II.

6. Most individuals stay on Stage I anywhere from three weeks to three months or more. The amount of yeast and the strength of the immune system do affect the overall time it takes to complete the program. These two variables cannot be measured accurately, only estimated. Some individuals stay on the entire program anywhere from two weeks to two years.

Stage One

Eat   Avoid

Grains

Amaranth

Eat	Avoid
flour	prepared flake cereals
whole	sprouted grain cereals

Barley

Eat	Avoid
flour	pearl
hatomugi	
(Japanese barley or Job's tears)	
whole	

Buckwheat

Eat	Avoid
flour	prepared flake cereals
groats	sprouted grain cereals
puffed cereal	

Corn

Eat	Avoid
blue corn meal, fine or course grind; undegerminated	blue corn meal, degerminated
cornmeal, fine or coarse grind; undegerminated	cornmeal, degerminated
masa harina	hominy grits
popcorn	prepared flake cereals
puffed cereal	sprouted grain cereals
	popcorn, microwave

Millet

Eat	Avoid
flour	prepared flake cereals
puffed cereal	
whole	

Eat	Avoid

Oats

Eat	Avoid
bran	granola
flakes	instant
flour	
groats	
quick cooking	
steel-cut, Irish or Scotch	

Quinoa

flour	
whole	

Rice

Eat	Avoid
basmati, brown	arborio
brown	basmati, white
(long, medium, or short grains)	brown, rice bran
quick, brown	cream of rice, white
puffed cereal	prepared flake cereals
rice, wild	sprouted grain cereals
texmati, brown	sushi rice
wehani	sweet, brown
whole grain baby cereal	texmati, white
	white
	(long, medium, or short grains)

Rye

Eat	Avoid
cream of rye cereal	prepared flake cereals
flour	sprouted grain cereals
groats	
puffed cereal	
whole grain baby cereal	

	Eat	**Avoid**

Spelt

Eat	Avoid
flour	prepared flake cereals
whole	sprouted grain cereals

Teff

Eat
flour
whole

Wheat

Eat	Avoid
berries	couscous
bran, unprocessed or miller's	cream of wheat (farina)
bulgur	farina
cracked	gluten flour
cream of whole grain cereal	prepared flake cereals
durum	processed baby cereal
graham flour	semolina
puffed, cereal	sprouted grain cereals
shredded, cereal	white flour
whole grain baby cereal	white pastry flour
whole wheat flour	
whole wheat pastry flour	

Pasta

Eat	Avoid
corn	bifun (Japanese noodles)
quinoa	farina
saifun (Japanese noodles)	semolina
soba (buckwheat)	somen (Japanese noodles)
udon (Japanese noodles)	white flour
whole wheat	

Cereals (see Grains)

Eat	Avoid

Baked/Prepared Products

Eat	Avoid
any whole grain unsweetened, unyeasted	any sweetened, yeasted chapatis, white flour
chapatis, whole wheat flour	mochi (sweet brown rice unleavened bread)
corn chips	
quick breads, unsweetened	pita bread
rice cakes or crackers, brown	potato chips
tortillas, corn or whole wheat	sourdough bread
	taro chips
	tortillas, white flour

Legumes

Eat	Avoid
beans and peas, canned (with water and salt only), dried, frozen	beans and peas, with sweetener or tomato sauce
black-eyed peas	bean sprouts, all kinds
chickpeas or garbanzo beans	peanuts
lentils	sweetened soymilk
soybeans	tempeh (fermented tofu)
soyflakes	tofu
soymilk, unsweetened	TVP (textured vegetable protein)
split peas	

Nuts and Seeds

This group of food may not be tolerated by those allergic to mold. If you have an allergy to mold, or if it is the mold season, avoid this section. If you can tolerate nuts and seeds, always put them into the oven for twenty minutes at 250 degrees to minimize the mold.

Eat	Avoid
almonds	coconut
Brazil	peanuts
cashews	pistachios
hazel	walnuts
macadamia	

Eat	**Avoid**

pecans
pinenuts
poppy
pumpkin
sesame (Tahini)
sunflower

Fruit

Eat	Avoid
fresh lemon, lime, eggplant (a half to a whole piece a day total)	all other fruits

Beverages

Eat	Avoid
juice, vegetable (no carrot or beet)	alcoholic drinks, all types
mugicha, toasted, whole barley	beet juice
coffee substitute, without malt	buttermilk
soy milk, unsweetened	carrot juice
Taheebo or Pau d' Arco Tea	chocolate drinks
water, plain or carbonated	coffee, regular or decaffeinated
	coffee substitutes (Pero)
	fruit juices, fresh or processed
	kefir
	milk
	soft drinks, sugared or diet
	sugar-sweetened drinks
	teas, any dried herbal, green, black, or oolong
	tomato juice
	V-8 juice

Eat	Avoid

Condiments and Seasonings

chicken broth,	capers, dried or powdered
without sweetener	garlic, dried or powdered
garlic, fresh only	herbs, dried or powdered
ginger, fresh only	ketchup
herbs, fresh only	miso (consolidated tofu soup)
lemon, one half per day	olives
onion, fresh only	onion, dried or powdered
pepper	pickles
salt	sauces with vinegar and
	sweetener (ketchup, steak sauce)
	sauerkraut
	spices, dried or powdered
	tomato sauce, fresh canned
	vinegar

Vegetables

vegetables, fresh, canned	cucumber skins
(except tomato), or frozen	mushrooms, all types
	potato skins
	soups prepared
	tomato, canned products

Proteins (animal)

antelope	antibiotics in meats and eggs
bear	(usually in beef, chicken, pork)
beef	meats, smoked and/or with
buffalo	sweetener (usually in prepared
caribou	meats)
chicken	
deer	
duck	
eggs	
elk	

Eat	Avoid
fish, all types	
frog legs	
game hen	
goat	
goose	
grouse (partridge)	
guinea fowl	
moose	
mutton	
peafowl	
pheasant	
pigeon (squab)	
pork	
quail	
turkey	

Dairy Products

Eat	Avoid
yogurt, plain with acidophilus culture	buttermilk
	cheese, all kinds
	cottage cheese
	kefir
	milk
	sour cream
	yogurt, with sweeteners

Stage Two Instructions

1. For the first three days of Stage II add only one new food from the Eat/Avoid list to your diet. The main areas to look at are: refined grains (like white flour), fruits, and fermented foods (vinegar, pickles) without sweetener. New foods are marked in bold italic.

2. Eat the chosen food for three days along with your regular Stage I foods. If no negative symptoms occur, continue eating that food and add another new food.

3. Remember to select only one food from a category at a time.

4. When adding fruit, eat no more than one serving a day. While working with the Symptom Chart (page 6) over the next three to six weeks, you can increase to two servings of fruit a day.

5. Choose low-carbohydrate selections when first adding fruit. See the Carbohydrate Value of Fruit (page 16).

6. Focus on your symptoms. Sometimes new symptoms (indigestion, gas) may occur from eating fruits or grains.

7. Do not eat fruit with your meal. For better digestion eat it at least an hour before or three hours after a meal.

8. If a symptom does occur or an existing one worsens from eating fruit, stop for four days, note how you feel and try it again. If your symptoms recur, stop eating fruit for two weeks, and try again. This rule for adding back fruit can be applied to any food. If it bothers you when you start eating it, stop and try again.

9. Do not eat moldy fruit of any kind, especially berries!

Stage Two

Eat   Avoid

Grains

Amaranth

Eat	Avoid
flour	prepared flake cereals
whole	sprouted grain cereals

Barley

flour
hatomugi
(Japanese barley or Job's tears)
pearl
whole

Buckwheat

Eat	Avoid
flour	prepared flake cereals
groats	sprouted grain cereals
puffed cereal	

Corn

Eat	Avoid
blue corn meal, fine or course grind; undegerminated and/or **degerminated**	prepared flake cereals
cornmeal, fine or coarse grind; undegerminated and/or **degerminated**	sprouted grain cereals
hominy grits	
masa harina	
popcorn, plain or **microwave,** without sweetener	
puffed cereal	

Eat	Avoid

Millet

Eat	Avoid
flour	prepared flake cereals
puffed cereal	
whole	

Oats

Eat	Avoid
bran	granola
flakes	
flour	
groats	
quick cooking or **instant,**	
no sweetener	
steel-cut, Irish or Scotch	

Quinoa

Eat
flour
whole

Rice

Eat	Avoid
arborio	prepared flake cereals
basmati, brown or **white**	sprouted grain cereals
brown (long, medium,	
or short grain)	
brown, rice bran	
cream of rice,	
whole or white	
puffed cereal	
quick, brown rice	
rice, wild	
sushi rice	
sweet, brown	
texmati, brown or white	
wehani rice	
white	
(long, medium, or short grain)	
whole grain baby cereal	

	Eat	Avoid

Rye

Eat	Avoid
cream of rye cereal	prepared flake cereals
flour	sprouted grain cereals
groats	
puffed cereal	
whole grain baby cereal	

Spelt

Eat	Avoid
flour	prepared flake cereals
whole	sprouted grain cereals

Teff

Eat	Avoid
flour	
whole	

Wheat

Eat	Avoid
berries	prepared flake cereals
bran, unprocessed or miller's	sprouted grain cereals
bulgur	
couscous	
cracked	
cream of wheat (farina)	
cream of whole grain cereal	
durum	
farina	
graham flour	
gluten flour	
puffed cereal	
semolina	
shredded cereal	
whole grain or **processed**	
baby cereal, without sweetener	
whole wheat or **white** flour	
whole wheat or **white**	
pastry flour	

Eat	Avoid

Pasta

bifun (Japanese noodles)
corn
farina
quinoa
saifun (Japanese noodles)
semolina
soba (buckwheat)
somen (Japanese noodles)
udon (Japanese noodles)
whole wheat or **white** flour

Cereals (see Grains)

Baked/Prepared Products

Eat	Avoid
any whole grain unsweetened, unyeasted	any sweetened or yeasted product
chapatis, whole wheat and/or **white flour**	mochi (sweet brown rice unleavened bread)
corn chips	pita bread
potato chips	sourdough bread
quick breads, unsweetened	
rice cakes or crackers, brown	
taro chips	
tortillas, corn, whole wheat, or **white flour**	

Legumes

Eat	Avoid
beans and peas, canned (with water and salt), dried, frozen	beans and peas, with sweetener or tomato sauce
bean sprouts, all kinds	peanuts
black-eyed peas	sweetened soymilk
chickpeas or garbanzo beans	
lentils	
soybeans	

Eat	**Avoid**

Eat
soyflakes
soymilk, unsweetened
split peas
tempeh (fermented tofu)
tofu
TVP (textured vegetable protein)

Nuts and Seeds

This group of food may not be tolerated by those allergic to mold. If you have an allergy to mold, or if it is the mold season, avoid this section. If you can tolerate nuts and seeds, always put them into the oven for twenty minutes at 250 degrees to minimize the mold.

Eat	Avoid
almonds	peanuts
Brazil	pistachios
cashews	walnuts
coconut, unsweetened, not dried	
hazel	
macadamia	
pecans	
pinenuts	
poppy	
pumpkin	
sesame (tahini)	
sunflower	

Fruit

Eat	Avoid
apple, all kinds	all dried fruit
applesauce, unsweetened	all fruit juice
apricot	grape
avocado	melon, all types
banana	raspberry
blackberry	

Eat	Avoid
blueberry	
boysenberry	
breadfruit	
cherry	
crabapple	
cranberry	
eggplant	
figs, fresh only	
gooseberry	
grapefruit	
guava	
kiwi	
kumquat	
lemon	
lime	
loganberry	
longberry	
loquat	
lychee	
Mandarin orange	
mango	
mulberry	
nectarine	
olallieberry	
orange	
papaya	
passionfruit	
peach	
pear	
persimmon	
pineapple	
plantain	
plum	
pomegranate	
pomelo	
prickly pear	

Eat	Avoid
quince	
strawberry	
tamarind	
tangelo	
tangerine	
tomato	

Beverages

Eat	Avoid
buttermilk	alcoholic drinks, all types
juice, **all vegetables**	cereal beverages
milk	chocolate drinks
Mugicha, toasted, whole barley	coffee, regular or decaffeinated
coffee substitute	fruit juices, fresh or processed
soy milk, unsweetened	kefir
Taheebo or Pau d' Arco Tea	soft drinks, sugared or diet
teas, any dried herbal,	sugar-sweetened drinks
Hoji-cha	teas, green, black, or
water, plain or carbonated	oolong (except Hoji-cha)
	tomato juice
	V-8 juice

Condiments and Seasonings

Eat	Avoid
capers	sauces with sweetener
chicken broth, without	(ketchup, steak sauce)
sweetener	tomato sauce, canned
garlic, fresh or **powdered**	
ginger, fresh or **powdered**	
herbs, fresh, **dried, or**	
powdered	
ketchup, without sweetener	
lemon, one half per day	
miso (consolidated tofu	
soup base)	
olives	
onion, fresh or **powdered**	

Eat	Avoid

pickles
pepper
salt
sauerkraut
spices, dried or powdered
tomato sauce, fresh
vinegar

Vegetables

vegetables, fresh, canned	cucumber skins
(except tomato) or frozen	mushrooms, all types
soups, prepared,	potato skins
without sweetener	tomato, canned products
(no tomato unless fresh)	

Proteins (animal)

antelope	antibiotics in meats and eggs
bear	(usually in beef, chicken, pork)
beef	meats prepared with sweetener
buffalo	
caribou	
chicken	
deer	
duck	
eggs	
elk	
fish, all types	
frog legs	
game hen	
goat	
goose	
grouse (partridge)	
guinea fowl	
meats, smoked	
moose	

Eat	Avoid

mutton
peafowl
pheasant
pigeon (squab)
pork
quail
turkey

Dairy Products

Eat	Avoid
buttermilk	cheese, all kinds
cottage cheese	kefir
milk	sour cream
yogurt, plain with	yogurt with sweetener
acidophilus culture	

Stage Three Instructions

1. For the first three days of Stage III add only one new food from the following Eat/Avoid list to your diet. The main areas to look at are mold family foods (baker's yeast, cheese, and mushrooms), walnuts, and melons. New foods are marked in bold italic.

2. Eat the chosen food for three days along with your regular Stage I and II foods. If no negative symptoms occur, continue eating that food and add another new food.

3. Remember to select only one food from a category at a time.

4. Eat no more than two servings of fruit a day.

5. When adding mold family foods (baker's yeast, brewer's yeast, cheese, and mushrooms) to your diet, start with only one mold family food. If you react, wait four days and try again. If you react again, wait for two weeks before trying again.

Stage Three

Eat   Avoid

Grains

Amaranth

Eat	Avoid
flour	prepared flake cereals
whole	sprouted grain cereals

Barley

flour
hatomugi (Japanese barley or
Jobs tears)
pearl
whole

Buckwheat

Eat	Avoid
flour	prepared flake cereals
groats	sprouted grain cereals
puffed cereal	

Corn

Eat	Avoid
blue corn meal, fine or coarse grind; undegerminated and/or degerminated	prepared flake cereals
cornmeal, fine or coarse grind; undegerminated and/or degerminated	sprouted grain cereals
hominy grits	
masa harina	
popcorn, plain or microwave, without sweetener	
puffed cereal	

Eat	Avoid

Millet

flour	prepared flake cereals
puffed cereal	
whole	

Oats

bran	granola
flakes	
flour	
groats	
quick cooking or instant, no sweetener	
steel-cut, Irish or Scotch	

Quinoa

| flour | |
| whole | |

Rice

arborio	prepared flake cereals
basmati, brown or white	sprouted grain cereals
brown (long, medium, or short grain)	
brown, rice bran	
cream of rice, whole or white	
quick, brown	
puffed cereal	
wild	
sushi rice	
sweet, brown	
texmati, brown or white	
wehani rice	
white (long, medium, or short grain)	
whole grain baby cereal	

Eat	Avoid

Rye

cream of rye cereal	prepared flake cereals
flour	sprouted grain cereals
groats	
puffed cereal	
whole grain baby cereal	

Spelt

flour	prepared flake cereals
whole	sprouted grain cereals

Teff

flour
whole

Wheat

berries	prepared flake cereals
bran, unprocessed or Miller's	sprouted grain cereals
bulgur	
couscous	
cracked	
cream of wheat (farina)	
cream of whole grain cereal	
durum	
farina	
graham flour	
gluten flour	
puffed, cereal	
semolina	
shredded, cereal	
whole grain or processed baby	
cereal, without sweetener	
whole wheat or white flour	
whole wheat or white pastry	
flour	

Eat   Avoid

Pasta

bifun (Japanese noodles)

corn

farina

quinoa

saifun (Japanese noodles)

semolina

soba (buckwheat)

somen (Japanese noodles)

udon (Japanese noodles)

whole wheat or white flour

Cereals (See Grains)

Baked/Prepared Products

any whole grain unsweetened, unyeasted or **yeasted bread**

chapatis, whole wheat flour or white flour

corn chips

mochi (sweet brown rice unleavened bread)

pita bread

potato chips

quick breads, unsweetened

rice cakes or crackers, brown

sourdough bread, unsweetened

taro chips

tortillas, corn, whole wheat or white flour

any yeasted sweetened product

Legumes

beans and peas, canned, dried, frozen or **with tomato sauce**

beans and peas, with sweetener

sweetened soymilk

Eat	Avoid

bean sprouts, all kinds
black-eyed peas
chickpeas or garbanzo beans
lentils
peanuts
soybeans
soyflakes
soymilk, unsweetened
split peas
tempeh (fermented tofu)
tofu
TVP (textured vegetable
protein)

Nuts and Seeds

This group of food may not be tolerated by those allergic to mold. If you
have an allergy to mold, or if it is the mold season, avoid this section. If you
can tolerate nuts and seeds, always put them into the oven for twenty minutes at 250 degrees to minimize the mold.

almonds
Brazil
cashews
coconut, unsweetened, not dried
hazel
macadamia
peanuts
pecans
pinenuts
pistachios
poppy
pumpkin
sesame (tahini)
sunflower
walnuts

Eat	Avoid

Fruit

Eat	Avoid
apple, all kinds	all dried fruit
applesauce	all fruit juices
apricot	
avocado	
banana	
blackberry	
blueberry	
boysenberry	
breadfruit	
cherry	
crabapple	
cranberry	
eggplant	
fig, fresh only	
gooseberry	
grapefruit	
grape	
guava	
jackfruit	
kiwi	
kumquat	
lemon	
lime	
loganberry	
longberry	
loquat	
lychee	
Mandarin orange	
mango	
melon, all types	
mulberry	
nectarine	
olallieberry	
orange	
papaya	

Eat	Avoid
passionfruit	
peach	
pear	
persimmon	
pineapple	
pitanga	
plantain	
plum	
pomegranate	
pomelo	
prickly pear	
quince	
raspberry	
strawberry	
tamarind	
tangelo	
tangerine	
tomato	

Beverages

Eat	Avoid
buttermilk	alcoholic drinks, all types
juice, all vegetables	cereal beverages
kefir	chocolate drinks
milk	coffee, regular or decaffeinated
Mugicha, toasted, whole barley	fruit juices, fresh or processed
"coffee" substitute	soft drinks, sugared or diet
soy milk, unsweetened	sugar-sweetened drinks
Taheebo or Pau d' Arco Tea	tea, black, or oolong
teas, any dried herbal, Hoji-cha	
or **green**	
tomato juice	
V-8 juice	
water, plain or carbonated	

Eat	Avoid

Condiments and Seasonings

Eat	Avoid
capers	sauces with sweetener
chicken broth, without sweetener	(ketchup, steak sauce)
	tomato sauce with sweetener
garlic, fresh or powdered	
ginger, fresh or powdered	
herbs, fresh, dried, or powdered	
ketchup, without sweetener	
lemon, one half per day	
miso (consolidated tofu soup base)	
olives	
onion, fresh or powdered	
pickles	
pepper	
salt	
sauerkraut	
spices, fresh, dried, or powdered	
tomato sauce, fresh or **canned, without sweetener**	
vinegar	

Vegetables

vegetables, fresh, canned, or frozen
cucumber skins
mushrooms, all types
potato skins
soups, prepared **without sweetener**
tomato, canned products, without sweetener

Proteins (animal)

antelope

Eat	Avoid
bear	antibiotics in meats and eggs
beef	(usually in beef, chicken, pork)
buffalo	meats prepared with sweetener
caribou	
chicken	
deer	
duck	
eggs	
elk	
fish, all types	
frog legs	
game hen	
goat	
goose	
grouse (partridge)	
guinea fowl	
meats, smoked	
moose	
mutton	
peafowl	
pheasant	
pigeon (squab)	
pork	
quail	
turkey	

Dairy Products

Eat	Avoid
buttermilk	yogurt, with sweetener
cottage cheese	
cheese, all kinds	
kefir	
milk	
sour cream	
yogurt, plain with acidophilus culture	

Maintenance for a Healthy Life

When most people start this diet, they are happy to know there is an end to it. But before returning to your old habits, remember these suggestions about staying healthy:

1. Use sweetener only on special occasions. Don't use them daily.

2. When selecting a sweetener, try molasses, honey, barley malt, rice syrup or maple syrup. These choices have more vitamins and minerals to offer than the empty calories of processed sugar.

3. If you've been given a course of antibiotics after a serious illness or medical emergency, stop using sweetener completely. Depending on how sick you are, you might start on Stage I again until you are feeling better. You don't want to give yeast a chance to get out of balance when your defenses are low.

4. Continue to take your acidophilus or bifidus daily as insurance that your Candida will stay in balance with your good bacteria.

5. Try to keep your fat intake below thirty percent of your total daily calories. Fat is the place where toxins are stored in the body, which can lead to health problems like cancer and heart disease.

6. Eat at least five servings of fruits and vegetables a day. The Tufts University Diet and Nutrition Letter defines a serving as: one cup of raw leafy greens; half a cup of other kinds of vegetables; one medium apple, orange, banana, or similar-size fruit; half a cup of small or diced fruit; one quarter-cup of dried fruit; three-quarters of a cup pure fruit or vegetable juice.

7. If you are a practicing vegetarian, which many health practitioners encourage, remember these guidelines for food combining:

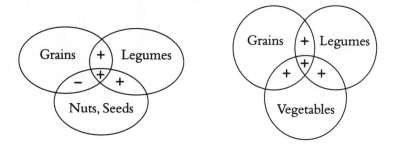

The + signs indicate a combination that is a complete protein and the − signs indicate one that isn't complete.

8. Remember that you truly are what you eat. Organic, fresh whole foods will offer you more nutrition than those which are processed and full of chemicals.

9. Your body is made up of ninety percent water. Drink eight glasses of purified (not distilled) water daily to help flush out toxins.

10. Now that you feel healthier and stronger, exercising for half an hour four to five times a week will insure that you'll feel this way for a long time. Whether it be cycling or dancing, the key to regular exercise is finding something that you enjoy doing.

Chapter Three

꧁

Candida Antifungal Preparations
and How They Work

I T'S THE SECOND or third day of using an antifungal medicine. Instead of feeling better, you feel horrible. What's going on?

You are experiencing what's called the "die-off" phase of a prescribed (or non-prescribed) medicine. Most antifungal medications or preparations inhibit the growth of new yeast buds. Some medications work locally while others work systemically, traveling through the blood supply to the whole body. During the initial phase of the program, the yeast cells die and produce toxic substances throughout the body. These toxins often cause headaches, joint pain, nausea, tiredness, and heavy night sweating. Die-off symptoms are most intense for the first three to four days of the medication process. Some individuals notice an increase of die-off symptoms at each increase of their dosage.

An antifungal program can be administered in two ways: with a prescription drug from a doctor, or with a series of supplements, herbs, or preparations from a health care practitioner (acupuncturist, chiropractor, or naturopath). This chapter will discuss the most common drugs and alternative preparations used for antifungal programs.

Your doctor or health practitioner should monitor your die-off symptoms so that your medication is not too stressful for you. If your die-off symptoms are extremely debilitating, the dosage is decreased and then slowly increased, or in some cases eliminated entirely. The quantity of intense symptoms varies according to an individual's health.

Even though you may initially feel worse, with perseverance and patience you will eventually feel better and be less symptomatic. Here are some things to do to make this difficult period easier on your body:

1. Exercise to speed oxygen to the cells and remove toxins. Work up a good sweat for at least twenty minutes, but don't overdo it. Try a nice long walk in clean air.

2. Drink at least two quarts or more of purified water daily to help to flush out toxins from the cells.

3. Get plenty of rest. Try to get eight hours of sleep per night, or take naps throughout the day.

4. Eat a well-balanced diet and don't skip meals. Feed your body all the nutrients it needs to overcome Candida. Take an all-inclusive vitamin and mineral supplement daily to balance your diet, along with extra vitamin C (a natural antihistamine).

5. During sleep, try to avoid exposure to items you have allergic reactions to (feathers, dust, mold, or cat hair) so that your immune system will be given the rest it needs to more vigorously eliminate the Candida. Prescription allergy treatments (shots or drops) will also strengthen your immune system.

6. Create as much of a stress-free environment as you can. Meditate, pray, or visualize yourself as a glowing picture of health again. Practice daily for thirty minutes putting your stresses into a state of suspension. *Countless studies have shown that any type of meditation can greatly increase overall performance and the ability to manage one's health.*

7. Start your medication so that the second and third days fall when you have a lighter schedule than usual (on the weekend, for example). Don't plan to start the Candida diet when

the stress of having to eat and socialize will be too over-whelming, both physically and emotionally. Socializing will be much easier after the initial two weeks of the program.

8. Die-off is very stressful to the body, which is often already overloaded with toxins from the air, water, and food we consume. Try relieving this overload by drinking grapefruit tea. Grapefruit tea is acidic while Candida and its wastes are alkaline. By drinking this tea you will help reverse the toxic excess alkaline that yeast produces.

To make the tea, wash an organic (if possible) grapefruit and cut it up into sections, while leaving on its skin. Place it in a nonmetallic pot with two pints of filtered water, cover and simmer for ten minutes. Let cool to room temperature with the lid on the pot, then pour through a sieve to filter out the grapefruit sections. Drink a couple of glasses a day to help with severe die-off symptoms.

9. When this period of die-off is over, reward yourself with some type of physical and/or emotional enjoyment that's not food. Get a friend or companion to share or help in finding a pleasing reward (flowers, a massage, or tickets to a concert). You deserve it.

Below are some of the most commonly used products physicians and alternative health practitioners use to eliminate Candida and strengthen the immune system.

Prescribed Antifungal Medications

Nystatin, USP (Mycostatin)

Nystatin is an antifungal medication developed some forty years ago from a mold that inhibits other molds from growing, including Candida albicans. Nystatin can be used as a cream, ointment, suppository, or taken orally in tablet and powder form. Orally, the usual adult dosage is from 1/16 teaspoon to ¼ teaspoon four times a day (qid) (⅛ tsp. equals 500,000 IUs). Nystatin has virtually no side effects with the exception of die-off symptoms. Nystatin works locally, not systemically in the blood. It goes through the digestive tract into the small and large intestines, gradually eliminating the Candida's overgrowth. Candida can live in all of the body's mucous membranes (in the mouth, sinuses, stomach, and intestines), but it primarily resides in the junction of the large and small intestines.

Depending upon the individual's problem and the doctor's approach, treatment with Nystatin can last from two months to two years. There's no way to pre-determine treatment time due to certain variables such as the health of your immune system, or whether you have allergies or an ongoing virus that you are constantly fighting.

If your doctor has prescribed Nystatin to be taken three or four times a day, it's important to do so routinely. Don't skip a dose and then later double-up on the amount (this could make you sick with too much die-off). Because of the way yeast grows, it's better to take the Nystatin consistently at regular intervals throughout the day.

The old saying "things get worse before they get better" is appropriate here. When you start taking Nystatin, the toxins of the dead yeast produce an alkaline environment which actually favors the growth of more yeast throughout the body. You may suddenly end up with thrush (oral Candida) or a vaginal yeast infection because of the alkaline environment so favorable to yeast growth. Some doctors recommend rinsing with Nystatin oral powder to control thrush (¼ teaspoon Nystatin powder in tepid water). Another product used for this problem is called Orithrush Gargle and Mouth Rinse by Cardiovascular Research (see page 186).

To prevent a mild vaginal yeast infection from getting worse, some doctors suggest douching with Nystatin powder, then two days later douching again with acidophilus powder (one teaspoon of either powder to one quart slightly tepid water). There are other effective douche preparations: Orithrush Douche by Cardiovascular Research; sorbic acid; vinegar; Pau d'Arco tea.

If you don't like to douche and have a mild infection, you can use acidophilus suppositories available from your health food store. Moderate to severe infections are usually treated by your doctor with Nystatin or Mycostatin suppositories or creams. If you are prone to yeast infections, try douching or using the acidophilus suppositories routinely through your ovulation cycle, when the yeast can become the most vaginally active.

Nizoral (Ketoconazole)

Nizoral is a broad-spectrum antifungal drug developed twelve years ago, and is taken orally once a day. In a small percentage of people, Nizoral produces serious side effects that cause liver enzymes to become depleted. If no history of liver problems is indicated, and the drug is used for more than three months, your doctor may monitor you with a blood test to make sure the liver enzymes are not being affected. Nizoral is absorbed into the bloodstream and becomes available systemically. It is also very effective in controlling vaginal yeast infections. Nizoral is often better tolerated than Nystatin because of how the die-off affects different people using each of these drugs.

Diflucan (Flucanazole)

Diflucan was first introduced in 1990 as a broad-spectrum antifungal drug. Diflucan works the same way as Nizoral in that it is absorbed into the blood. Physicians have found Diflucan to be even more effective than Nizoral in controlling yeast infections in shorter periods of time, and without the same effect on the liver enzymes. However, it is much more expensive at $10 to $12 per pill (Nizoral costs approximately $1 per pill).

Non-Prescription Antifungal Preparations

Australian Tea Tree Oil

This preparation comes from the leaves of a tree in Australia which possesses germicidal, fungicidal, and antiseptic properties. The manufacturers of Australian Tea Tree Oil claim that it is nontoxic and nonirritating to normal tissue. It can be found in a variety of preparations ranging from toothpaste for thrush to a topical oil for yeast on the skin or scalp. It can be used to treat Candida on the surface of the skin or in the mouth while taking some other form of antifungal preparation orally.

Caprylic Acid

Caprylic acid is a saturated fatty acid effective in treating yeast over-growth in the intestinal tract. It is manufactured by several companies with various brand names (Mycopryl 680, Caprystatin, Caprinex, Candistat, Kaprycidin-A, Capricin, and Capralin). Some of these brands work in the lower intestines or stomach only, while others work throughout the entire digestive tract. No serious side effects are noted with the use of this antifungal substance. However, caprylic acid does cause die-off symptoms. Some individuals report digestive upsets with its use. It is good to have a doctor or health care practitioner monitor your symptoms when using caprylic acid. Amounts vary with different manufacturers, but are generally between 300–600 milligrams a day.

Cantrol

Cantrol is a nutritional approach to controlling Candida, combining acidophilus, Pau d'Arco, a hypoallergenic antioxidant, linseed oil, and citrus seed extract. One may experience die-off using this product because of Pau d'Arco and the citrus seed extract. Cantrol is distributed by Nature's Way (see page 187).

Citrus Seed Extracts

Citrus seed extract is a broad-spectrum antifungal product derived from the extracts of tropical plants. It is produced and distributed by various companies under various product names (ParaMicrocidin, Paracan 144, DF100, Citricidal, and Seed-a-Sept-II). Citrus seed extract manufacturer's claim that it has no specific toxicity except that it can cause burning of the mouth if not diluted properly in water. Citrus seed extract can cause die-off for some individuals.

Garlic

Taking garlic can improve one's health in so many ways, from suppressing cholesterol synthesis to reducing blood clots, from stimulating the immune system to combating the growth of yeast. Garlic stimulates the immune system to kill yeast and thereby prevents the yeast from spreading further. At the First World Congress on the Health Significance of Garlic and Garlic Constituents in 1990, researchers showed that garlic does not have to be consumed raw to be effective. Also, the odor and freshness of garlic are not critical to its overall benefits. The aged, deodorized forms of garlic in capsules or cooked garlic have been reported to work better than fresh garlic, which is harder to digest. Garlic may cause die-off symptoms.

Pau d'Arco (Bow Stick, LaPacho, Taheebo, Ipe Roxo, Quaw Bark, Tecoma)

Pau d'Arco is an antifungal made from tree bark. It comes in either capsule form or as a tea. In the tea form, most practitioners recommend at least two cups a day, and in the tablet form, it varies from each manufacturer. Some women have reported using Pau d'Arco as a successful douche for vaginal yeast infections. Pau d'Arco may cause die-off symptoms.

Acidophilus

Acidophilus, the group of friendly bacteria that includes lactobacillus acidophilus, lactobacillus bifidus, streptococcus faecium, and other bifido bacteria, replenishes the good bacteria in your intestinal tract. Acidophilus is found in yogurt and also in concentrated powder or capsule form. Acidophilus fights off microbes, synthesizes B vitamins, contributes to the body's immune cells, aids in digestion, prevents the fungus form of Candida albicans from forming invasive germ tubes in the colon, and impedes the growth of Candida in the digestive tract and vagina.

All of the waste products in the body are acidic and acidophilus ("acid loving") helps to eliminate the body's waste. When acidophilus is depleted by antibiotics, poor diet, and stress, Candida moves in. Candida then produces alkaline waste products which our bodies are not able to eliminate. To correct this destructive imbalance, you must replace intestinal acidophilus. For anyone on an antifungal program, taking an acidophilus supplement or eating lots of yogurt with active cultures, can be one of the most effective parts of a daily routine.

There are many versions of acidophilus products to choose from. You can find acidophilus at health food stores or through mail order vitamin companies (see page 185). Some manufacturers separate the lactobacillus acidophilus and bifidus into separate jars, while others combine them. As to what works best, you will have to choose, but remember these important things while you are shopping for good products:

Use a powder that has a high count of good bacteria (four to ten billion organisms). Mix in tepid water (never hot) and drink during or after a meal when your stomach is less acidic.

Get a product that has been refrigerated in a dark bottle and keep it cold, without excessive moisture; temperatures above 78 degrees can destroy the acidophilus bacteria. Avoid heat treated products, as heat kills this live culture.

Always check for an expiration date on the acidophilus product or yogurt. Don't let it linger too long in your refrigerator.

Avoid products that contain sweeteners.

Acidophilus products are made from cow's milk but a less allergenic product can be made with a different medium like carrots. Ask for allergy-free products if you are allergic to milk.

If and when you can drink milk again, provide your good bacteria with its favorite food, lactose (milk sugar).

Tanalbit™

Tanalbit consists of natural tannins that are naturally antifungal when combined with zinc. Along with managing yeast overgrowth in the intestines, it can help with acute and chronic diarrhea, colitis, constipation and spastic colon. The manufacturers of Tanalbit claim that it has few side effects, especially if it is taken with meals. This product is produced by Scientific Consulting Service (see page 188).

Nutritional Supplements, Digestive Enzymes, and Immune-Supportive Products

This section describes some of the nutritional supplements and herbs most commonly used by doctors and health practitioners for treatment of Candida. Most of these items help aid the body in its fight against yeast and supply the necessary nutrients for a treatment program.

Nutritional Supplements

Ideally it is best to get your vitamins and minerals from the food you eat. But with the daily restrictions of time, diet, and availability, you should take supplements as a practical alternative. If you use a vitamin/mineral product, find one that is yeast-free and contains similar amounts of the following nutrients:

Vitamins

Vitamin A	10,000 IUs
Beta-carotene	15,000 IUs
Bioflavonoids	250 mg.
*Biotin	1000 mcg.
Vitamin C	1000–3000 mg.
Cobalamin (B$_{12}$)	50 mcg.
Vitamin D	200–400 IUs
Vitamin E	300–600 IUs
Folic acid	400–800 mcg.
Vitamin K	50–300 mcg.
Niacinamide (B$_3$)	25–100 mg.
Pantothenic acid (B$_5$)	50–150 mg.
*Pyridoxine (B$_6$)	50–75 mg.
Pyridoxal-5-phosphate	50 mg.
Riboflavin (B$_2$)	25–75 mg
Thiamine (B$_1$)	50–75 mg.

★ These nutrients are often increased because of Candida and/or PMS symptoms.

Minerals

Calcium	800–1000 mg.
Chromium	200–500 mcg.
Copper	2 mg.
Iodine	150–225 mcg.
Iron	10–18 mg.
*Magnesium	400–800 mg.
Manganese	5–10 mg.
Molybdenum	500 mcg.
Selenium	200–300 mcg.
Zinc	15–30 mg.

All nutritional supplements should be taken after you eat, never on an empty stomach.

Magnesium, a mineral, and B_6, a member of the B-complex family, are two nutrients that are depleted by the yeast's consumption of food and are often used to reverse PMS symptoms.

Biotin, also a member of the B-complex family, is the only vitamin required by Candida for its growth. Paradoxically, Biotin prevents the conversion of yeast into a fungus in the intestines. The fungus could create holes which allow food particles into the blood stream causing the immune system to react allergically. This theory, suggested by Jeffrey Bland, Ph.D., explains the need for adequate Biotin supplementation.

The extra supplementation of magnesium, B_6, and Biotin can help control the yeast, as well as offer other benefits of a balanced multiple vitamin/mineral program.

Digestive Enzymes

Enzymes allow the body to digest food. The stomach, pancreas, and liver are the main places in the body that use enzymes. There is a limited supply of enzymes and they decrease with age, stress, and

---

* These nutrients are often increased because of Candida and/or PMS symptoms.

illness. Although enzymes are found abundantly in fresh, unprocessed, natural foods, they are easily destroyed by temperatures over 120 degrees Fahrenheit (49 degrees Celcius). A lack of enzymes is indicated when you are not digesting your food as well as you could and problems such as bloating and gas occur. This is why many health practioners suggest the use of digestive enzymes during a Candida program.

There are two types of digestive enzymes that can be taken as supplements. The first type consists of essential enzymes to aid the stomach in digesting protein. These enzymes are most commonly found in two tropical fruits: *bromelain* from pineapple and *papain* from papaya. The second type, pancreatic enzymes, helps the pancreas by supplying necessary glandular support. The pancreas secretes lipases, amylases, and proteases which are found in pancreatic enzymes. Excessive enzyme production, often due to Candida, weakens the pancreas. Many practitioners think that pancreatic insufficiency is the cause of several degenerative diseases. Research is being done using pancreatic enzymes to help reverse cancer.

Both types of digestive enzymes should be taken during or just after a meal. They often prevent the problem of digestion from getting worse, while assisting the stomach or pancreas. They can usually be found in health food stores, or try ordering through Scientific Consulting Service (page 188). Digestive enzymes are not suggested for use when there is inflammation of the stomach lining.

Immune-Supportive Products

Coenzyme Q_{10} (Co Q_{10}, Ubiquinone)

Coenzyme Q_{10} is an electron carrier important to many body energy systems, stimulating the immune system, helping circulation, and aiding metabolic function. Many doctors and other health practitioners suggest Coenzyme Q_{10} for combating chronic infections, including Candida, AIDS, and Chronic Fatigue Syndrome. Coenzyme Q_{10} is found in oily fish, organ meats, and grains, but is also available in capsules or drops.

Germanium

Germanium is a trace element found in soil as well as certain foods and herbs. In 1967 Kazuhiko Asai isolated a compound (GE 132) from Germanium that he spent the next fifteen years researching. GE 132 enhances the immune system by stimulating interferon production and macrophage and lymphocyte activity. GE 132 may also suppress cancerous tumor activity. It enriches oxygen in the body, which helps prevent disease. GE 132 has been used extensively for resisting Candida's growth by stimulating the immune system.

Echinacea

Echinacea root stimulates the immune system while purifying blood and lymph systems. Studies have shown that echinacea root can increase white blood count and stimulate the lymphatic system to clear waste material. It is recommended that this herb (two to four capsules a day) be used for no more than three to four weeks at a time because of possible liver irritation or changes in normal intestinal flora.

Golden Seal

Golden Seal root is an antibacterial, antiseptic, detoxifier, and antiparasitic herb. Like echinacea, it is generally used for only short treatment periods (two to three weeks) to prevent irritation to the liver. It helps stimulate the immune system to resist the growth of Candida.

Ultra Balance

Ultra Balance, a powder that you mix in water, nourishes the body and consists of several ingredients that cleanse the colon (where most of the Candida lives). Ultra Balance helps to rebuild the colon's cellular walls so that the "good bacteria" can grow again and take Candida's place. A synergized, oligoantigenic formula developed by Jeff Bland, this drink has the necessary vitamins, minerals, and selective food sources for friendly bacteria. It immediately goes to work on the cellular repair necessary to correct the yeast problem. It can also be used as part of an elimination program for food sensitivity investigations. This formula is distributed through Metagenics (see page 187).

Essential Fatty Acids

Essential fatty acids are polyunsaturated fatty acids that include linoleic, linolenic, and arachidonic. Essential fatty acids cannot be manufactured by the body but are very important to several bodily functions. Flax seed (linseed), rapeseed (canola), sunflower, safflower, corn, evening primrose, and borage are essential fatty acids (EFAs) found in plants. EFAs are also found in the fat of cold-water fish like salmon, mackerel, sardines, tuna, and herring. Being diverse, EFAs can help with eczema, arthritis, heart disease, and PMS. They are required for the cellular structure of all cells and membranes. Many doctors and health practitioners recommend EFAs to manage Candida, allergies, and PMS.

Chapter Four

✿

The Social Side of Your Recovery

ENERGY LEVELS DURING Candida can vary enormously. Most of the information in this chapter applies to those whose energy is low. For those with adequate energy, skip to the section on Eating Out Successfully.

Support Groups

Patients low on energy should without hesitation or embarrassment seek help in support groups. Local hospital or county health departments have listings of support groups. These groups hold meetings where participants focus on giving each other information and help. If a meeting drains your energy, change groups. If meetings are taken over by professional complainers, go elsewhere. Stick to groups sparked by new information and where you feel the glow of support. A good support group should leave you feeling invigorated and confident about your recovery. Write the International Health Foundation, Inc., Post Office Box 3494, Jackson, Tennessee 38303 for more information.

Chronic Fatigue groups can also be very helpful; the issues involved are much the same. Write The CFIDS Association, Inc., Post Office Box 220398, Charlotte, North Carolina 28222 for their newsletter, *The CFIDS Chronicle*.

Asking for Help

After years of talking with clients, Maureen has learned that the hardest part of any recovery is having to ask for help. When national columnist Judith (Miss Manners) Martin, was consulted on the problem said she had no magic answers. We say just ask. Even the slightest bit of help from others can be instrumental to your Candida recovery.

If your pitch to get help at a family meeting or at a table full of friends is unsuccessful, don't give up. Ask for help one-to-one. Keep in mind that your recovery will take some months and that you don't necessarily look sick. The best approach is to proceed in a matter-of-fact way, much in the way you would for recycling, car maintenance, watering the plants, or feeding the pets. Organize yourself, or if you have a family, organize them and delegate tasks. Be clear, calm, and banish any guilt you might be harboring.

What many patients appreciate is:

> Help with grocery shopping
>
> Special cooking
>
> A modest exercise program with a friend
>
> Transportation to doctors, hair appointments, movies, or massage

If anyone asks if they can help, take up the offer immediately. A friend or family member could prepare packages of herbs (Foxy Herbs page 98), or cook brown rice (page 130) and bag it for the freezer, or make a special bread (pages 88, 90) or Almond Milk (page 96), or have a whole meal delivered.

Massages, shampoos, a trip to a restaurant or the movies are all welcome. It is both polite and smart to give your helper a choice of task . . . but don't turn down the offer.

Grocery Shopping

First, make a grocery list from the Eat/Avoid list for your stage and locate a store that carries the basic items you need. Second, locate a store that delivers if you are lacking energy. Any delivery charge will be worth the energy you will save shopping. Locate a meat department that carries organic meats or will order them for you. Show the Mail Order Food Sources (page 189) to a butcher who wants to help you. A little charm and humor go a long way in this department.

Cooking

Start by relieving your muscles. Back strain can be dramatically reduced by placing one foot up on a low stool (professional cooks do this). Cook sitting down when you can. Get a counter-high stool with a back rest (this could be a gift from a friend).

Maureen has heard countless complaints about the difficulty of cooking for the needs of both the Candida patient and the family. Making one staple grain for everyone is a start (polenta or brown rice). Add already prepared meat or fish, vegetables and salad, and provide pourable sauces and condiments for the rest of the family. If you work and must do the cooking as well, plan a series of meals, cook ahead, and freeze for later use.

Eating Out Successfully

Eating out can be quite a challenge for a Candida patient. One of Helen's best coping strategies was to make a nearby Chinese restaurant her once-a-week home. The maitre d' would greet her with: "Oh, yes! Shrimp, no soy, no MSG, no sugar, with garlic, brown rice. This way please!"

In general, Chinese and Iranian restaurants are best for your needs. Chinese cooks are wonderful about making dishes to order, and Iranians are strong on naturally whole foods like rice and vegetables along with plain, grilled shish-kabob. They often include grilled eggplant and peppers. In standard American restaurants, order plain meat or fish (without sauce), a salad with no dressing, and plain steamed or grilled vegetables (with butter only). Pour Your Salad Dressing (page 101) on the salad, whip out your own Whole Wheat Rolls (page 91), order bottled water, and you've got a respectable meal with very little fuss. In Stage II, you may add vinegar, tomatoes, and other items to your diet which will eliminate the need for planning and toting.

In fast food restaurants you can order almost nothing, sorry to say. After an extensive study of their complete ingredients list (they even put sugar in French fries), we found only one item to recommend: the garden or side salad without dressing!

Section Two

Recipes
for the Candida Diet

Chapter Five

❧

Eating Well with Candida

ACANDIDA DIET DOESN'T have to be bland, just careful. The following pages include recipes for fish, rice, eggs, vegetables, yogurt, garlic, and ginger. You'll find hot drinks, breads without yeast, several kinds of pancakes, crêpes, cereals, lots of interesting egg recipes, and even a milk substitute to put on your whole grain cereal.

The collection of recipes is definitely unbalanced—in favor of breakfast and portable lunches you can take to work, the hardest part of the diet. Your yeast, tucked away in the cozy darkness, doesn't know or care about breakfast, lunch, and dinner. Feed yourself on a diet free of the strictures of ordinary eating: the familiar eggs for breakfast, something light for lunch, something substantial for dinner. Our recipes will help you make the leap.

All the recipes start on Stage I, with the exception of a couple that begin on Stage II (Avocado Snack, Rosie's Posie Pasta). Many of our recipes are progressive, showing you how to add foods in Stage II and III.

Don't worry about esoteric groceries for the diet. You can buy everything you need to get well in an ordinary super market. For the truly adventurous, the Food List in chapter fourteen gives a complete listing of allowed foods. However, the foods found in our recipes are more than sufficient for your return to health. The recipes are intentionally kept simple so that you may add the allowed foods in the appropriate stages, but only as you desire. Teff flour and xanthum gum are the only mail order items to make a some yeast-free breads. The Mail Order Food Sources (page 189) will give you some options but these are the only ones actually needed.

It's a limited diet, but you can get well on this simple fare. If you want to explore further in the book, please do! There are combinations waiting to be discovered—and you may even have a company dinner or two! One is especially created for us by Julia Child. Other food luminaries have also contributed so there's no need to feel out of the mainstream. In fact, many of these recipes are distinctly glamorous. The diet is a clean and healthy one. In California, many perfectly healthy women and men eat this way simply because it's wise to do so: there's nothing wrong with them at all.

Naturally, we have a list of "watch-out-for."

1. Make your food choices (meat, poultry, eggs) free of antibiotics whenever possible. Antibiotics also exist in cow's milk, so use it in moderation. Soy milk is antibiotic-free.

2. Buy "organic" vegetables and fruits. This word is a giant catch-all, but in general, use unsprayed vegetables and fruits. Ask the produce manager at your grocery store.

3. Use filtered water, and carry it with you wherever you go. The most reliable source comes from your own water filter at home. For the best choices refer to *Consumers Report* February 1993, or National Sanitation Foundation (NSF) at 3745 Plymouth Road, Ann Arbor, Michigan 48105, or call (313) 769–8010. You can also contact the EPA's Safe Drinking Water Hotline (800) 426–4791. Ask for their free booklet "Is your Drinking Water Safe?"

4. For food storage: to avoid mold that can grow in food even if it can't be seen, refrigerate food covered *for two to three days only.* For frozen foods, the general rule is no more than two weeks, tightly sealed.

5. It's always sensible to keep the fat content of any diet as low as possible. We've been fairly lavish with oils and butter because often the new Candida patient needs the calories to gain or maintain weight. But generally speaking, healthy diets are low in fat and so is this one. Adjust recipes to your own needs. If oil is reduced, increase the liquid in the recipe to maintain the balance. Use oil in a spray can and/or a Teflon pan.

6. When we mention "oil or spray for the pan," we mean any cold-pressed vegetable oil (safflower or olive). For the spray, we prefer olive oil.

7. Use of artificial sweeteners is tempting but dangerous. If used at all (and we don't recommend *any*) use only very small amounts, and sparingly. Almond Milk (page 96) will help as a comforting flavoring.

8. When a recipe asks for plain yogurt, buy yogurt with live cultures or ingredients such as lacto-bacillus acidophilus and lacto-bacillus bifidus. Avoid yogurts that have sweeteners and fruit.

9. Candida diet patients have to read labels carefully. Most crisp breads do not contain yeast, but some do. Practice your label reading skills on them. Be careful! Malted barley, rice syrup, dextrose, monoglycerides, diglycerides, and malt flavor are all sugars.

10. Since breakfast is the hardest (most non-traditional) meal for the new Candida patient, it's easy to latch onto a favorite recipe and eat it every day. Please do not do this! This method could jeopardize a speedy recovery.

Don't be intimidated by this list—do the best you can and don't make you life more complicated. *Occasional errors will not be important to your overall recovery.*

The most important point of this introduction is to shake loose that part of the brain that categorizes food into the familiar breakfast, lunch, and dinner. Try soup for breakfast and eggs for dinner.

Eating creatively is the key. Keep yourself fed and the yeast unhappy and deprived, is our advice.

In New York City, Garrison Keillor enjoys the escape from routine midwestern thinking. He admires New Yorkers who have the courage and imagination to " . . . eat ice cream for breakfast." In this same vein we say, be different and eat popcorn for breakfast.

The following meal plans can be made using both the recipes from the book as well as foods listed in the stages. Any complete meal plan is a suggestion for using several different items in that particular stage. Eat a daily balanced diet of whole grains, vegetables, fruits, dairy products and, if so inclined, meat. We hope that these suggestions will inspire your creativity to keep expanding your daily meal plan.

Suggested Meal Plan for Stage I

Breakfast
Oven-Coddled Eggs (page 124) or any egg recipe (pages 125, 126)
Whole Wheat Bread (page 90), toasted, with butter
Ginger Tea (page 98) or Herbal Infusions (page 99)

Lunch
Make-Ahead Protein Salad (page 105)
Senate Bean Soup (page 109)
Corn tortillas
Ginger Tea (page 98) or Herbal Infusions (page 99)

Dinner
Basic Brown Rice (page 130)
Peel and Eat Shrimp (page 142)
Steamed assorted vegetables (carrots, broccoli, green beans)
Ginger Tea (page 98) or Herbal Infusions (page 99)
Lick That Lemon! (page 99)

Snack
Chip and Nut Butter Snack (page 97)
Whole shelled almonds
Cut vegetables (carrots, broccoli, cauliflower, jicama)
Celery sticks with almond butter

Suggested Meal Plan for Stage II

Breakfast
Back to Bed Popovers (page 84) with
Warmed Fruit Purée (page 101), strawberry or any other fresh
    fruit in season
Any egg recipe (pages 124–126)
Ginger Tea (page 98) or Herbal Infusions (page 99)

Lunch
Basic Tuna Sandwich (page 141) with mayonnaise instead of
    yogurt on
Whole Wheat Bread (page 90)
Cut vegetables (carrots, broccoli, cauliflower, jicama) with
Plain low fat yogurt with dried herbs (dill and tarragon) and
    dried garlic dip
Ginger Tea (page 98) or Herbal Infusions (page 99)

Dinner
Company Chicken (page 138) with whole mustard seeds
Three Stage Cole Slaw (page 106)
Old Fashioned Baked Potato (page 118)
Steamed assorted vegetables (carrots, broccoli, green beans)
plain mineral water with lemon slice

Snack
Celery sticks with almond butter
Avocado Snack (page 96)

Suggested Meal Plan For Stage III
Breakfast
Yeasted Whole Grain Bread (without sweetener), toasted, with
    butter
Scrambled eggs with cheese
Herbal Infusions (page 99)

Lunch
Jennifer's Soup (page 108) with canned, unsweetened tomato paste
Yeasted, unsweetened crackers
Pick-Me-Up Trout Snack (page 100)

Dinner
Brown Rice and Toasted Nuts with Creamy Polenta (page 131)
    with walnuts
Chicken with Roasted Red Peppers (page 138)

Snack
Melon slices
Celery sticks with unsweetened peanut butter
Avocado Snack (page 96)

Suggested Meal Plan for a Special Occasion — Stage I
Breakfast
Tiny Russian Pancakes (Blini), with yogurt and caviar (page 89)
Ginger Tea (page 98) or Herbal Infusions (page 99)

Lunch
Marion Cunningham's Winter Vegetable Cobbler (page 117)
Ginger Tea (page 98) or Herbal Infusions (page 99)

Dinner
Julia Child's Special Dinner (page 145)
plain mineral water with lemon slice or
Ginger Tea (page 98) or Herbal Infusions (page 99)

Hors d'Oeuvres
Garlic Inspiration (page 97) with crispbreads or
Marinated Yogurt Cheese (page 113) with plain rice cakes

Suggested Meal Plan for Special Occasion — Stage II
Breakfast
Yogurt Crêpes (page 91) with
Warmed Fruit Purée (page 101), strawberry or any other fresh
    fruit
Herbal Infusions (page 99)

Lunch
Rosie's Versatile Vegetable Ragoût (page 118) with tomatoes
Teff Bread (page 88) with
Marinated Yogurt Cheese (page 113) with dried herbs

Dinner
Wolfgang Puck's Bay Scallops (page 144) with apples
Basic Brown Rice (page 130)
Basic Green Salad (page 105) with Your Salad Dressing (page 101)

Hors d'Oeuvres
Avocado Snack (page 96) with corn chips

Suggested Meal Plan for Special Occasion — Stage III
Breakfast
Protein Waffles (page 87) topped with walnut pieces and
Warmed Fruit Purée (page 101), strawberry or any other fresh fruit
    in season
Herbal Infusions (page 99)

Lunch
Warm Chicken Salad (page 107) with walnut pieces
Dorothy's Flaky Whole Wheat Biscuits (page 86)
Narsai's Mother's Summer Drink (page 113)

Dinner
Julia Child's Special Dinner (page 145) with vinegar substitute for
    lemon juice
plain mineral water with lemon slice

Hors d'Oeuvres
Melon slices
Celery sticks with unsweetened peanut butter
Avocado Snack (page 96) with yeasted, unsweetened crackers

Suggested Meal Plan for Vegetarians — Stage I

Breakfast
Night Before Oatmeal (page 123) topped with Almond Milk
    (page 96)
Ginger Tea (page 98)
Brown Rice Flour Soda Bread (page 84), toasted, with butter

Lunch
Delicious Eggplant "Bread"(page 86)
Make Ahead Protein Salad (page 105)
Cucumber Refresher (page 111)
Ginger Tea (page 98) or Herbal Infusions (page 99)

Dinner
Dayna's Stand By Dinner (page 116)
Steamed assorted vegetables (carrots, broccoli, green beans)
Dorothy's Flaky Whole Wheat Biscuits (page 86) with butter
Ginger Tea (page 98) or Herbal Infusions (page 99)

Snack
Chip and Nut Butter Snack (page 97)
Whole shelled almonds
Cut vegetables (carrots, broccoli, cauliflower, jicama)

Suggested Meal Plan for Vegetarians — Stage II

Breakfast
Hot Corn Cereal (page 132)
Almond Milk (page 96)

Lunch
Anni's Garbanzo Rice Fiesta Salad (page 104) with tomatoes
Teff Bread (page 88)
Steamed assorted vegetables (beets, broccoli, green beans)
Ginger Tea (page 98) or Herbal Infusions (page 99)

Dinner
Tofu Steaks and Brown Rice (page 119) with soy sauce
Three Stage Cole Slaw (page 106)
Steamed assorted vegetables (carrots, broccoli, green beans)
Ginger Tea (page 98) or Herbal Infusions (page 99)

Snack
Avocado Snack (page 96)
Chip and Nut Butter Snack (page 97)
Whole shelled almonds
Cut vegetables (carrots, broccoli, cauliflower, jicama)

Suggested Meal Plan for Vegetarians — Stage III

Breakfast
Puffed Grain Cereal With Walnuts (page 123)
Teff Bread (page 88) toasted, with butter
Ginger Tea (page 98) or Herbal Infusions (page 99)

Lunch
Rosie's Posie Pasta (page 133) with grated cheese
Teff Bread (page 88)
Ginger Tea (page 98) or Herbal Infusions (page 99)

Dinner
Tofu Steaks and Brown Rice (page 119) with sautéed mushrooms
Three Stage Cole Slaw (page 106)
Whole Wheat Rolls (page 91)
Ginger Tea (page 98) or Herbal Infusions (page 9)

Snack
Melon slices or apple slices with peanut butter
Avocado Snack (page 96)
Chip and Nut Butter Snack (page 97)
Whole shelled almonds
Cut vegetables (carrots, broccoli, cauliflower, jicama)

Suggested Meal Plan for Vegetarians Special Occasion — Stage I

Breakfast
Charles Shere's Bog Man Cereal (page 122)
Brown Rice Flour Soda Bread (page 84) toasted, with butter
Ginger Tea (page 98) or Herbal Infusions (page 99)

Lunch
Old-Fashioned Baked Potato (page 118), topped with Narsai
    David's Versatile Savory Sauce (page 99)
Alice Waters' Salad for Fanny (page 104)
Ginger Tea (page 98) or Herbal Infusions (page 99)

Dinner
Marion Cunningham's Winter Vegetable Cobbler (page 117)
Cucumber Refresher (page 111)
Brown Rice Flour Soda Bread (page 84)

Hors d'Oeuvres
Garlic Inspiration (page 97) with crispbreads or
Marinated Yogurt Cheese (page 113) with plain rice cakes

Suggested Meal Plan for Vegetarians Special Occasion — Stage II

Breakfast
Yogurt Pancakes (page 92) topped with almond slivers and
Warmed Fruit Purée (page 101), strawberry or any other fresh
    fruit in season
Ginger Tea (page 98) or Herbal Infusions (page 99)

Lunch
Rosie's Versatile Vegetable Ragout (page 118) with tomatoes
Whole Wheat Bread (pages 90)
Cut vegetables (carrots, broccoli, cauliflower, jicama)
Ginger Tea (page 98) or Herbal Infusions (page 99)

Dinner
Rosie's Posie Pasta (page 113) with tomatoes
Carrot and Leek Side Dish (page 115)
Basic Green Salad (page 105) with Your Salad Dressing (page 101)
plain mineral water with lemon slice
Fruit Fool (page 112)

Hors d'Oeuvres
Apple slices or carrot sticks with almond butter
Chip and Nut Butter Snack (page 97)
Garlic Inspiration (page 97) with crispbreads or
Marinated Yogurt Cheese (page 113) with plain rice cakes

Suggested Meal Plan for Vegetarians Special Occasion — Stage III

Breakfast
Yogurt Crêpes (page 92) with fresh fruit and walnuts
Ginger Tea (page 98) or Herbal Infusions (page 99)

Lunch
Seated Garlic Pasta (page 134)
Cut vegetables (carrots, broccoli, cauliflower, jicama)
Ginger Tea (page 98) or Herbal Infusions (page 99)

Dinner
Wild Rice Soup (page 111)
Three Stage Cole Slaw (page 106) with fruit
Basic Green Salad (page 105) with Your Salad Dressing (page 101)
Narsai's Mother's Summer Drink (page 113)

Hors d'Oeuvres
Garlic Inspiration (page 97) with yeasted, unsweetened crackers or
Marinated Yogurt Cheese (page 113) with plain rice cakes

Chapter Six

❧

Breads and Baked Goods

W HAT WE WOULDN'T have given for these recipes years ago! It's amazing how you miss bread if you can't have it. Helen will never forget her first taste of a bread her Candida diet didn't forbid: it was a whole wheat and rye bread leavened with airborne wild yeast and it took four to five days for the bread to rise.

It's much easier to make your own tasty bread at home! You will find nearly a dozen bready things to eat here. Jackie Mallorca, noted food writer and associate writer with James Beard in his later years, created many of these recipes (Teff Bread, Whole Wheat Bread, Whole Wheat Rolls, Yogurt Crêpes, and Yogurt Pancakes). Her contribution is the most valuable for the bread-starved Candida patient.

Back to Bed Popovers
Brown Rice Flour Soda Bread
Delicious Eggplant "Bread"
Dorothy's Flaky Whole Wheat Biscuits
Protein Waffle
Jackie Breads and Others
   Teff Bread
   Tiny Russian Pancakes (Blini)
   Whole Wheat Bread

Whole Wheat Rolls
Yogurt Crêpes
Yogurt Pancakes

Back to Bed Popovers

These easy-to-make popovers are great for breakfast and go well with any soup or stew. If you can get someone to slip them into a cold oven, you have only to get out of bed once to turn the heat down, and then you can enjoy them half an hour later. These are great by themselves and even better with Warmed Fruit Purée (page 101). Unlike other recipes, this one starts at Stage II.

Serves 1 to 2

Stage II
olive oil spray for greasing cups
2 eggs
¾ cup plain yogurt
1 cup unbleached flour
1 tablespoon melted butter
¼ teaspoon salt

Lightly oil five 6-ounce custard cups or a heavy popover pan. In a medium bowl, beat eggs well with yogurt. Add flour, butter, and salt and beat again. The batter should be very thin. If necessary, add a tablespoon or two of tepid water so that mixture pours easily. Fill cups ⅔ full; if using custard cups, place on a rigid baking sheet. Slide into a cold oven and bake at 450 degrees for 25 minutes. Without opening oven door, reduce heat to 350 degrees and bake 35 minutes longer. Remove from oven and pierce popovers to let steam escape. Serve with Warmed Fruit Purée.

Brown Rice Flour Soda Bread

One of Ireland's great culinary legacies, soda bread can be prepared in less than ten minutes and bakes in half an hour. In this version, brown rice flour and nutty-tasting rice bran give it a special grain-filled fragrance and goodness. Making this bread in four small loaves vastly improves the texture.

Have all the ingredients and utensils ready before you start mixing: when alkaline baking soda and acid yogurt combine, the soda bread must be baked as soon as possible. If you linger, the bread won't rise properly. Measure the ingredients carefully to insure consistent results.

Rice flour, rice bran, and xanthan gum powder (a natural carbohydrate derived from corn) are available at natural food stores or order from Bob's Red Mill (page 189). Xanthan is essential for a springy, bread-like texture not otherwise attainable when baking with brown rice flour. The tablespoon of molasses (usually a forbidden ingredient) is a very small amount and makes for a delicious and pleasing bread.

Makes four 5-ounce loaves

Stage I
    1½ cups (7 ounces), brown rice flour
    ½ cup (1½ ounces) rice bran
    ½ cup (1½ ounces) cornstarch
    1 teaspoon kosher or sea salt
    2 teaspoons xanthan gum powder
    1 teaspoon baking soda
    1 large egg
    1 cup plain low fat or nonfat yogurt
    1 tablespoon molasses

Place baking sheet in oven and preheat to 425 degrees. In a large mixing bowl, sift together the flour, bran, cornstarch, salt, xanthan, and baking soda. Discard any chaff remaining in sifter. In a separate bowl, beat together the egg, yogurt, and molasses. Pour liquid ingredients over flour mixture and mix with rubber spatula. Gather dough and turn out onto a lightly floured work surface. Form into a four small balls. Dust a wide metal spatula and set the balls on it. Dust the balls with rice flour and cut a cross from one side to the other with a sharp knife. Slide dough from the metal spatula onto the baking sheet in the oven. Bake for 30 minutes and let cool on rack.

Delicious Eggplant "Bread"

Helen discovered this when she was ravenous for bread and took up one of the eggplant slices she had made for her family. Eggplant could be called "the great pretender." It can masquerade as a meat substitute and as a "bread" for sandwiches with tomatoes and mozzarella cheese (Stage III). Even better, eggplant can be baked with olive oil and used with soups and stews (any Stage). Don't be shy in trying eggplant—this is a tasty treat. See below for two methods of preparation.

Serves 2

Stage I
>   one eggplant
>   oil for the pan
>   salt and pepper to taste

Peel and cut eggplant crosswise into ⅓-inch rounds.

To sauté: In a heavy frying pan, heat 1 to 3 tablespoons of olive oil or spray pan with oil before heating. Heat pan over medium-high heat and add eggplant slices, browning both sides to your taste. Add more olive oil if slices stick to the pan.

To bake: Lightly brush slices with olive oil and bake at 350 degrees in a heavy frying pan or baking sheet for 15 minutes. Season with salt and pepper to taste. Eat just like bread!

Dorothy's Flaky Whole Wheat Biscuits

Dorothy Calimeris is one of those professional bakers who can look at a recipe and tell you instantly how it will turn out. In thirty seconds she translated a favorite biscuit recipe using white flour into one we could use, and never dropped a flake along the way.

Makes 8 to 9 biscuits

Stage I

> 2 cups whole wheat pastry flour
>
> 1 teaspoon baking powder
>
> 2 teaspoons baking soda
>
> pinch of salt
>
> ⅓ to ¼ cup vegetable shortening
>
> ½ cup yogurt and ½ cup water mixed together

Preheat oven to 425 degrees. In a large mixing bowl, combine all dry ingredients using your hands or a fork. Stir and toss until all ingredients are well mixed. With floured hands, break shortening into 5 or 6 chunks and add to dry ingredients. Lightly rub the flour and shortening together, reaching down to the bottom of the bowl to get all the flour mixture. When the mixture resembles bread crumbs, add the yogurt and water mixture all at once. Stir the mixture together—it will be a sticky mass of dough. Do not overmix! Scoop it out of the bowl and put it on a lightly floured work surface.

Wash and dry your hands, then re-flour them. Knead the dough 10 times and form into a circle about 9 inches around and ¾ inch thick. Cut biscuits with a 2-inch cookie cutter, and place on a lightly greased cookie sheet. Bake for 12 to 15 minutes or until biscuits are nicely golden on top. Serve warm with lots of butter.

Protein Waffle

This lovely waffle batter can also be used for pancakes. The recipe is easily doubled and makes an elegant Sunday brunch. It is Maureen's weekly family treat. Serve with Almond Milk, or top with plain yogurt and chopped, toasted almonds. Leftover waffles or pancakes can be eaten later as bread.

Makes 1 waffle or pancake

Stage I

> oil for the waffle iron
>
> 2 eggs
>
> ⅔ cup plain yogurt
>
> ½ cup uncooked rolled oats

⅛ teaspoon salt
optional toppings:
extra plain yogurt
Almond Milk (page 96)
chopped and toasted almonds

Brush or spray waffle iron with olive oil. Heat waffle iron on medium heat. Using a blender, combine eggs, yogurt, rolled oats and salt on blend for five seconds. (Consistency of yogurt may vary. Just be sure you have a pourable batter.) Spoon the batter onto the iron, spreading with the back of the spoon to the edge so that batter is about ¼-inch thick and entirely covers the metal. Close iron, then check occasionally for doneness. This waffle will not spread. Cook until the top turns a reddish pecan color. Serve on a warmed plate and top with plain yogurt, Almond Milk, and/or almonds.

Jackie Breads and Others

When Jackie Mallorca was diagnosed wheat intolerant, she set to creating some very eatable breads. Appalled by the terrible substitutes for wheat products she found on the market, she invented Teff Bread (see following recipe) and invited an old friend, Chuck Williams founder of Williams/Sonoma to tea. After a slice or two, Mr. Williams commented, "Hmm, delicious," and asked about the recipe. Now that's a compliment! Jackie takes two or three rolls tucked into an airtight plastic bag with her when she dines out. This conversation piece gives her healthy and complete nutrition. People are genuinely impressed with her ingenuity and the charming way she takes care of herself. There's no need for her to apologize for her condition. We all admire people who take care of themselves.

Teff Bread

This nutty-tasting, close-textured brown bread is good with sweet butter. Unlike commercially made breads, it contains no preservatives, so should be enjoyed when fresh. You can also slice the loaf and store individual servings in the freezer, in airtight plastic bags.

Makes one 20-ounce loaf or ten 2-ounce rolls

Stage I
    1 cup teff flour
    1 cup whole wheat flour
    4 teaspoons baking powder
    ½ teaspoon salt
    3 large eggs
    ½ cup plain yogurt
    ¼ cup water
    2 tablespoons vegetable oil

Preheat oven to 350 degrees. Sift flours, baking powder, and salt into a large mixing bowl. In a separate bowl, combine eggs, yogurt, water, and vegetable oil. Beat well. Pour liquid ingredients over dry ingredients and mix well with a wooden spoon. Oil an 8- by 4-inch loaf pan. Transfer batter to the loaf pan and smooth top. Bake for 60 minutes, then turn out onto a rack to cool. To make rolls, divide batter into ten equal portions and place in muffin cups lined with paper cupcake liners. Bake for 45 minutes, then turn out onto a rack to cool.

Stage II
Add 1 teaspoon anise seeds or sesame seeds on top of bread in pan before baking.

Tiny Russian Pancakes (Blini)

Like many things in life, these get better and better with time. The batter will keep for two to three days covered in the refrigerator. Blini are good with Ginger Tea (page 98) and go well with Salmon Soup (page 110). You can build a little party around these pancakes. They are filling without being heavy and were often used at post-ballet midnight suppers in old Russia, topped with sour cream and caviar.

Serves 1 (about twenty 3-inch pancakes)

Stage I
>2 eggs
>1 cup buckwheat flour
>1 teaspoon baking powder
>⅛ teaspoon soda
>½ teaspoon salt
>½ cup water
>½ cup yogurt
>oil for the pan
>*optional toppings:*
>butter or yogurt
>caviar

In a medium bowl, lightly beat eggs. Add dry ingredients and mix. In a separate bowl mix together water and yogurt. Add yogurt mixture and mix vigorously. Brush or spray a heavy frying pan with olive oil, then set pan on high heat. When pan is very hot, pour small spoonfuls (about one tablespoon) of the batter into the pan. Let the pancakes cook for a minute, until the edges are crisp and the surface has little bubbles. Turn heat down to medium-low and turn pancakes over. Cook the second side for a bit longer. When pancake holds together on a spatula, it's done.

Serve with butter or yogurt on top, with a spot of caviar.

Whole Wheat Bread

This dense whole grain loaf is quick to prepare and has a very tempting aroma when it comes out of the oven. Store any leftovers in an airtight plastic bag in the freezer because this type of bread dries out quickly.

Makes one 12-ounce loaf

Stage I
>1 cup whole wheat flour
>½ cup teff flour
>2 teaspoons baking powder
>½ teaspoons salt

2 large eggs
¼ cup water
2 tablespoons vegetable oil
1 teaspoon poppy seeds (optional)

Preheat oven to 425 degrees. Sift flours, baking powder, and salt into a large mixing bowl. In a separate bowl, beat eggs lightly. Pour off and reserve two tablespoons for brushing top of loaf. Add water and vegetable oil to beaten eggs. Pour liquid ingredients over flour mixture and stir well to make a smooth dough. Turn out dough onto a lightly floured surface and pat into a ball, handling as lightly as possible. Roll into a log twelve inches long. Place log on an oiled baking sheet or lined with baking parchment. Add a few drops of water to reserved beaten egg and brush over loaf. Sprinkle with poppy seeds. Make several diagonal slashes across loaf and bake for 35 minutes. Cool on a wire rack.

Whole Wheat Rolls

Makes six 2-ounce rolls

Proceed as above, but cut the log into six equal pieces. Form each into a flat round and place on baking sheet. Brush tips with reserved egg and sprinkle with poppy seeds. Bake for 20 minutes. Serve warm, or allow to cool and freeze in individual airtight plastic bags for convenient "carry along" purposes.

Yogurt Crêpes

These thin French-style pancakes are delicious rolled up with a savory filling and served hot, or used like tortillas. To freeze, interleave the crêpes with plastic wrap or waxed paper, and wrap airtight.

Makes approximately ten crêpes.

Stage I
½ cup teff flour
⅓ cup cornstarch

pinch salt
3 large eggs
½ cup yogurt
½ cup water
2 tablespoons butter

Combine teff flour, cornstarch, and salt in a large mixing bowl. In a separate bowl, combine and beat together eggs, yogurt, and water. Melt butter in an 8½-inch iron frying pan and allow it to brown. Add browned butter to liquid ingredients, and pour over the flour mixture. Mix well with a fork, adding a little more water if batter is too thick to pour easily. Reheat pan (grease with a little more butter from time to time), and pour in ¼ cup batter. Tilt pan to cover bottom with batter. Cook over medium-high heat for 45 seconds or until lightly browned. Loosen edges of crêpe with a metal spatula and turn to cook the other side about 30 seconds. Repeat with remaining batter, stacking crêpes on a plate.

Yogurt Pancakes

Cooking pancakes without butter or oil in a nonstick skillet gives them an excellent surface texture. These little griddle cakes are good served cold and spread with butter.

Makes about twenty 3-inch round pancakes

Stage I
⅔ cup teff or buckwheat flour
⅓ cup cornstarch
1 teaspoon baking powder
pinch salt
1 large egg
2 tablespoons vegetable oil
½ plain yogurt
½ cup water

Stage II
Add ¼ teaspoons nutmeg or cinnamon to batter.

Sift teff flour, cornstarch, baking powder, and salt into a bowl. In a separate bowl combine egg, vegetable oil, yogurt, and water. Pour liquid ingredients over dry ingredients and mix well. Heat a non-stick skillet over medium heat. Pour 2 tablespoons of batter for each pancake into pan, making three or four at a time. Cook 90 seconds on both sides, or until golden brown.

Chapter Seven

Mavericks

Here's a collection of little ideas and tips that are a category by themselves. They are all useful for rounding out your diet. The word "maverick," comes from a Texas cattleman named Maverick who refused to brand his herd. If any cows were found without a brand, they were called, "mavericks."

A favorite in this section is the very satisfying and highly caloric Chip and Nut Butter Snack, still enjoyed in post-Candida times. Don't overlook the hint called Lick That Lemon! It makes your mouth feel fresh after a heavy meal and reduces the desire for dessert.

Almond Milk
Avocado Snack
Chip and Nut Butter Snack
Garlic Inspiration (Baked White Garlic)
Ginger Tea
Foxy Herbs
Herbal Infusions
Lick That Lemon!
Narsai David's Versatile Savory Sauce
Pick-Me-Up Trout Snack
Toasted Nuts
Warm Fruit Purée
Your Salad Dressing

Almond Milk

This delicately flavored milk is a great addition to many foods. It brings competing flavors into a state of détente—sort of the Henry Kissinger of the Candida diet. It's good on cereal and as a topping for waffles and pancakes. Made thickly, it can be used as a spread or a thickener for soup. The ratio of almonds to water varies in our recipe to allow you to choose between a spread or milk-like consistency.

> Stage I
> 1 cup almonds, whole, freshly roasted
> 2¼ to 4 cups water

Place the almonds and water (2¼ cups for topping or spread, 4 cups for drinking) in a tightly closed jar and store in the refrigerator for 1 to 2 days at the most. Pour into a blender and blend until the mixture is smooth. To use it as a drink, strain first. The remaining almond paste is delicious and can be tossed on cereal, vegetables or rice.

Avocado Snack

This delightful little snack can also double as an almost lunch. Serve with your favorite bean or corn chips. Add a little fresh lemon juice to your favorite drinking water, and relax. Because avocados are actually a fruit, this is a Stage II recipe.

> Serves 1 to 2

> Stage II
> 1 to 2 avocados
> fresh lemon juice
> salt to taste

Scrub and pare the avocados as you would an apple. With another knife, scrape the newly exposed dark green surface. (The second knife removes any mold carried onto the avocado by the first knife.) Cut the avocado in half lengthwise, remove pit, and slice each half into several wedges. Arrange avocado slices or halves on a plate. Drizzle with lemon juice and salt lightly.

Chip and Nut Butter Snack

This is one of the best little suggestions in the book. When an absolutely instant quick fix is needed, this is it.

> Stage I
>> whole grain chips (corn, brown rice, bean, or any
>> combination)
>> almond butter

Dip whole grain chip into almond butter. Enjoy with your favorite ice cold drinking water.

Garlic Inspiration (Baked White Garlic)

Baked garlic is one of the most satisfying dishes imaginable. Squeeze cloves of baked garlic onto Teff or Whole Wheat Bread to transform any simple soup dinner into something special. Alice Waters made this dish famous at the Chez Panisse Garlic Festival in 1974. Our version is tamer but still wonderful.

> Serves 2 to 3

> Stage I
>> olive oil
>> 2 to 3 whole heads of new garlic
>> salt and pepper to taste
>> butter (optional)
>> any fresh herbs, Provençal mixture preferred

Preheat oven to 250 degrees. Pick off and brush away loose outer skins of garlic heads. Cloves should not come apart. Pour ¼ inch of olive oil into a small shallow baking dish. Add whole heads of garlic, root side down. Sprinkle with salt and pepper. Dot with butter, if desired. Add a few sprigs of any fresh herb or herb mixture. Bake uncovered 1½ hours, spooning over a bit of olive oil at the end of baking time. Spread over bread (buttered if desired) and serve at any meal.

Ginger Tea

This popular tea can be enjoyed any time of day. It soothes indigestion, helps with flatulence, and aids circulation. You can make it as strong or as weak as you like.

Serves 1

    1 cubic inch fresh ginger root, peeled and cut into small pieces

    boiling water (use fresh cold water to start)

Pour boiling water over ginger pieces in your cup or mug and let stand for 10 to 20 minutes or until desired strength. Experience will guide you to the length of steeping time.

Foxy Herbs

This wonderful idea contributed by our redoubtable recipe editor, Anne Fox, is from the 1950s. Keep a small juice canister packed with fresh home grown herbs, cut-up frozen, and ready for use. This is an easy task that a friend can do for you.

Stage I

    6 bunches green onions

    or

    2 small bunches parsley

    or   all yielding approximately

    1 large ginger root   one cup

    or

    3 bunches of chives

Wash and dry fresh herbs, then chop coarsely. Take an empty large juice concentrate can and cut off the ends. Put the chopped herbs into the container and double wrap tightly using plastic wrap. Place in a airtight plastic bag and freeze.

When you want some herbs, unwrap and push through the

amount desired, cut off what you need, re-wrap and return to the freezer.

Herbal Infusions

Finding the following fresh herbs for teas or herbal infusions is a favor you might consider asking of a friend.

Serves 1

Stage I

> Chamomile—good for relaxation and as a sleeping aid.
> Mint—good for digestion.
> Thyme—excellent to boost nasal passages and chest
>   during a cold.

For freshly cut, delicately flavored herbs a small fistful is required. For older, stronger tasting herbs a smaller amount will do but a longer steeping time is required. A little experimentation will be your guide. Place the herbs in a clean tea pot and pour boiling water over the herbs. Water that has not quite come to the boil yields slightly mellower flavor.

Steep for a few minutes or as long as desired.

Lick That Lemon!

So often after a heavy meal, you long for the fresh and clean taste of fruit. When that happens, simply cut a lemon in half and lick it. The bit of acid in the lemon will not hurt you, and the dividend is a fresh-feeling mouth.

We know of no better method for cleaning and refreshing the mouth and for reducing the longing for a sweet dessert. Try it!

Narsai David's Versatile Savory Sauce

An Old-Fashioned Baked Potato (page 118) is happy to be topped by this sauce, as are vegetables. It may be added to yogurt as a spread on rice cakes or crispbreads. This sauce can also be wonderfully embellished by a teaspoon of butter.

Serves 1 to 2

Stage I

> 1 onion, coarsely chopped
>
> 6 to 8 cloves garlic, peeled
>
> 1 cup canned chicken or vegetable broth

Preheat oven to 350 degrees. Lay onion and whole garlic cloves in a small casserole. Pour broth over all and bake uncovered for about half an hour, or until onion is soft. When done, spoon into a blender and purée for several seconds. Pour into a warmed bowl and serve.

Pick-Me-Up Trout Snack

A welcome crunchy protein snack can be put together easily with any leftover cooked fish.

Serves 1 to 2

Stage I

> 1 cooked (grilled, fried, or steamed) trout
>
> 4 to 5 crispbread or whole grain crackers
>
> ¼ cup plain yogurt
>
> 1 heaping tablespoon whole mustard seed, or fresh dill weed, chopped
>
> 1 lemon, halved

Skin, bone, and flake the cooked fish. Place on crackers. Mix yogurt and mustard seed or dill weed, then gently spread over fish. Drizzle lemon juice over all.

Toasted Nuts

Experience has proven that this is the best formula for roasting nuts.

Serves 1

Stage I

> 1 cup of nuts (almonds, Brazil, cashews, hazel, pecans, pine nuts, sesame)

Preheat oven to 250 degrees. Chop nuts, if desired. Sprinkle nuts on an ungreased cookie sheet. Bake 20 to 25 minutes.

Warm Fruit Purée

After you've passed Stage I, here's a way to welcome delicious fruits back into your diet.

Serves 1 to 2

Stage II
  ¾ cup strawberries, peaches, or nectarines

If using berries, carefully wash and stem them. Roughly cut fruit into halves or chunks. Blend on medium speed in blender or chop finely by hand. Place in a small frying pan on medium and cook long enough to warm fruit. Pour over pancakes or cereal for a well-earned treat.

Your Salad Dressing

Double or triple this recipe, store in a tightly covered jar in the refrigerator and you are ready to go out at a moment's notice. This is also good with Three Stage Cole Slaw (page 106).

Serves 1 or 2

Stage I
  ¼ cup lemon juice
  ¾ cup olive oil
  salt and pepper to taste
  garlic, fresh pressed, to taste
  fresh-cut herbs to taste
  glass jar (bigger than 8-ounces) with lid

Stage II
  Substitute ¼ cup rice or regular vinegar for lemon juice.

Place ingredients in jar, fasten lid tightly, and shake vigorously.

Chapter Eight

Salads, Soups, and Yogurt

OUPS AND SALADS can be enjoyed any time of day. Warm or fresh salads can be carried anywhere in lidded containers. The Warm Scallop Salad with Ginger is a particular favorite of ours. If you think you don't like soup, try nuzzling up to these recipes. Soup can be the best breakfast food there is for the Candida-challenged—hot, sustaining, and constantly varying. These are specific recipes, but don't forget that almost any leftover meat or vegetable is delicious when dropped into a homemade chicken broth. (Making broth is another good task for a friend who wants to help you.)

Yogurt has been around for centuries and makes a refreshing accompaniment to many meals. A dollop of yogurt on top of any stew or soup adds a nice contrast in temperature and flavor. Narsai's Mother's Summer Drink or Soup is highly recommended. It can make a simple sandwich lunch seem lavish.

Salads
Alice Waters' Salad for Fanny
Anni's Garbanzo Rice Fiesta Salad
Basic Green Salad
Make-Ahead Protein Salad
Three Stage Cole Slaw
Warm Chicken Salad
Warm Scallop Salad with Ginger

Soups
Jennifer's Soup
Salmon Soup
Senate Bean Soup
Short-Order Soup
Wild Rice Soup

Yogurt
Cucumber Refresher Salad/Dessert (Raita)
Easy Cheese
Fruit Fool
Marinated Yogurt Cheese
Narsai's Mother's Summer Drink or Soup

Alice Waters' Salad for Fanny

Great ideas cross time and space to meet in unexpected ways. One day on the spur of the moment, Alice Waters of Chez Panisse made up a simple and delicious salad for her six-year-old daughter, Fanny. In that moment, East and West came together—Alice's salad was very much like the classic created in 1940 by the famous Japanese healer, Hawayo Takata, who went from house to house cooking for her patients and supervising their recovery. If we could only have visiting nurses like that today!

Serve 1 to 6

Stage I
½ cup grated celery, jicama, and carrots for each serving
lemon juice to taste

Layer each vegetable separately, one on top of the other, in a shallow dish. Squeeze a little lemon juice on top.

Anni's Garbanzo Rice Fiesta Salad

Maureen's friend Anni Amberger-Warren, a wonderful Bay Area caterer, created this complete and tasty salad. This is a great one to make ahead of time.

Serves 3 to 4

Stage I
    1 15-ounce can garbanzo beans
    2 cups wild rice, cooked
    3 scallions, chopped fine
    ½ cup parsley, chopped
    1 teaspoon fresh jalapeño peppers, chopped fine
    salt and pepper to taste

Dressing
    juice from 1 large lemon
    ⅛ cup olive oil
    1 garlic clove, minced

Mix beans, rice, scallions, parsley, and peppers. Add salt and pepper to taste. Squeeze lemon juice on top. Combine olive oil with garlic and pour over all.

Basic Green Salad

Romaine, butter, red leaf, and iceberg lettuce (or any combination) can make terrific salads. Jicama, carrots, radishes, and turnips make excellent additions.
    Serves 2

Stage I, II, III
    3 cups washed lettuce leaves
    1 cup of pared and cut jicama, carrots, radishes, and/or
       turnips
    Your Salad Dressing (page 101)

Tear the lettuce leaves into bite-sized chunks and place in a large mixing bowl. Add cut vegetables and dressing. Toss lightly and serve.

Make-Ahead Protein Salad

This wonderful little meal is great to have on hand in the refrigerator and is very portable. It should be kept no more than two or three days.
    Serves 1 to 2

Stage I

    1 cup bulgur wheat

    2 cups boiling water

    1 bunch whole scallions, diced

    1 cup chopped parsley

    2 sprigs chopped mint

    2 tablespoons olive oil

    3 to 6 tablespoons lemon juice, to taste

    salt and pepper

Stage II

    2 cups diced tomatoes

Add bulgur wheat to boiling water, stir, reduce heat, cover and let simmer for 20 minutes. The bulgur wheat should be fluffy when done. Toss cooked bulgur wheat in bowl with remaining ingredients, adding lemon juice, salt, and pepper to taste. If desired, add diced tomatoes in Stage II. Serve with a dollop of plain yogurt and Delicious Eggplant "Bread" (page 86).

Three Stage Cole Slaw

Always tasty and popular, cole slaw is one of those versatile meal extenders. The following recipe is basic and tasty, especially with a bit of fresh lemon and freshly ground black pepper on top.

    Serves 2 to 3

Stage I

    3 cups green cabbage

    1 large carrot

    1 lemon

    black pepper

Rough cut the cabbage into strips, then bite-sized pieces. Place cabbage in a large mixing bowl and grate carrot directly into the bowl. Halve the lemon and squeeze juice over all. Toss and serve with pepper to taste.

Stage II
Add two tablespoons of rice vinegar and four tablespoons of lowfat mayonnaise. Mix thoroughly.

Stage III
To the above, add ¾ cup of pineapple chunks, fresh grapes, pomegranate seeds, grapefruit sections, or apple slices.

Warm Chicken Salad

The word "delicious" will have new meaning when you eat this interesting salad.

Serves 1

Stage I
    2 tablespoons almonds
    1 chicken breast with bone
    1½ cups cold water
    2 garlic cloves, minced
    ½ onion, chopped
    salt to taste
    3 to 4 leaves of lettuce
    lemon or lime juice
    ½ cup plain yogurt
    1 scallion, sliced

Stage II
    garnish with pomegranate seeds

Preheat oven to 250 degrees. Toast almonds on ungreased baking sheet in oven for 20 minutes. Remove and set aside to cool. In a medium pot combine chicken, water, garlic, onion, and salt to taste. Bring to a fast boil for 5 minutes, then lower heat and simmer uncovered for 30 minutes. Gather up cooled almonds in a tea towel, and roughly crush with a rolling pin. While still in the pot, roughly shred chicken away from bone using two forks and lay on lettuce-lined plate.

Sprinkle chicken with lemon or lime juice. Add a dollop of yogurt and garnish with crushed almonds, and scallions.

Warm Scallop Salad with Ginger

Try this simple yet quickly made salad for an elegant lunch or supper. The recipe can easily be doubled or tripled. Anne Fox was enthusiastic when served this salad at a tasting session and took the recipe home with her to make a treat for her husband.
Serves 1

Stage I
     1 cup Basic Brown Rice (page 130)
     ⅓ pound bay or regular scallops cut into quarters
     oil for the pan
     2-inch piece peeled fresh ginger
     1 clove garlic, peeled (optional)
     1 lemon
     several leaves butter lettuce

Cook rice ahead of time. It will remain warm for about 20 minutes and the scallops only take only a few minutes to cook. Spray cold frying pan with oil before heating or heat a large frying pan to medium-high heat and add enough oil to cover bottom of the pan. Add scallops. As scallops begin to sauté, shred ginger and garlic directly onto scallops. Squeeze ½ lemon over scallops. Stir scallops for 3 minutes, until they look firmer than when you started. Do not overcook. Scallops are at their best when tender. Arrange scallops in nest of lettuce, garnish with half a lemon sliced into wedges. Spoon juices over the rice and serve.

Jennifer's Soup

Jennifer, of Brooklyn New York by way of Trinidad, is one of those natural cooks who can make soup out of whatever is in the refrigerator. This half-hour soup for Stage III tastes like more than the sum of its parts.
Serves 4

Stage III

> 8 cups water
> 4 to 6 red potatoes
> 5 to 6 carrots
> 2 yellow onions
> 1 green pepper
> 2 stalks of celery
> 2 cloves garlic, minced
> 4 tablespoons tomato paste
> ¼ teaspoon each paprika, garlic, and onion powder
> 1 teaspoon, or more of butter
> salt and fresh ground pepper, to taste

Boil water in 5-quart pot, then lower to simmer. Chop and dice the vegetables and add to pot. Add garlic, tomato paste, seasonings, and butter. Simmer covered for 30 minutes. Salt and pepper to taste, then serve.

Salmon Soup

This elegant little soup takes minutes to prepare and is a lovely accompaniment with Tiny Russian Pancakes.

Serves 2

Stage I

> 1 8-ounce can chicken broth
> 1 filet (5 ounces) salmon, flaked or chopped, cooked steak
> 3 scallions, sliced
> few sprigs parsley, chopped
> half a lemon
> 1 recipe Tiny Russian Pancakes (page 89)
>
> *optional garnish*
> plain yogurt
> caviar

In a medium saucepan, simmer broth for about 3 minutes. Continue to simmer broth as you add salmon, scallions, parsley, and juice of half a lemon. Let soup continue to simmer while you make Tiny Russian Pancakes, about 15 minutes. Serve soup with pancakes on a side plate. Garnish with plain yogurt. For company, add a dab of caviar to each pancake.

Senate Bean Soup

There's almost a century of tradition behind this hearty soup, which is served daily at U. S. Senate dining room. It's our favorite as well. No politics involved, just plain good taste. We both love this for breakfast.

Serves 4 to 6

Stage I
>   5 cups water
>   1 cup (½ pound) navy or white beans, washed
>   1 whole lean pork chop, (5 ounces)
>   1 large onion, roughly chopped
>   salt and pepper to taste

Put all ingredients into a 3 quart pot, bring to a boil, reduce to a simmer, and cover. Stir occasionally. Cook 3 to 4 hours until meat falls from the bone. Shred meat with two forks into soup and be sure to discard all bones. Salt and pepper to taste.

Short-Order Soup

Quickly made soups that don't require a lot of time at the stove are always a favorite. Here's the quickest Helen has dreamed up, with a satisfying, homemade taste.

Serves 1 to 2

Stage I
>   2 8-ounce cans of chicken or vegetable broth
>   1 large leek, or small bunch of scallions

Pour broth into medium saucepan on low heat. Slice leek or

scallions lengthwise. Cut off most of the green, rinse thoroughly, then snip into crosswise slices (scissors can help). Add to soup and simmer for 10 minutes.

Wild Rice Soup

Wild rice is very flavorful and good for you. Once cooked and frozen, it's perfect to add to a simple soup like this one. Tiny Russian Pancakes (page 89) are good with this.

Serves 2 to 4

Stage I

2 cups cooked wild rice

32-ounce can of chicken or vegetable broth

4 ounces canned salmon

lemon juice to taste

Simmer all ingredients together for no more than 20 minutes. Sprinkle lemon juice on top before serving.

Cucumber Refresher Salad/Dessert (Raita)

The easiest dessert and/or salad to make in the first stage of the diet is a famous Middle Eastern dish known as raita in India. You could call it "Godsend Salad" because after a wholesome, savory meal of meats and rice, it takes the place of fruit. Use it with mint, garlic and cucumber for a salad; with mint only for dessert.

Serves 2

Stage I

1 cup plain yogurt

½ cup peeled, chopped cucumber

½ teaspoon fresh minced garlic

½ teaspoon of salt

For dessert

1 cup plain yogurt

1 tablespoon minced fresh mint

Finely chop the cucumber. In a medium mixing bowl, add cucumber to the yogurt with the garlic and salt. Mix all ingredients together. When making raita as a dessert, finely mince the fresh mint leaves. Both will keep for 2 to 3 days.

Easy Cheese

Yogurt cheese is indeed easy. It's so versatile you'll want to have it in your refrigerator all the time. Use it plain, marinated as in the recipe below, or add such tidbits as almonds, salmon, and chopped fresh vegetables.

Serves 4

Stage I

> 32 ounces plain yogurt, regular or nonfat
> cheesecloth (double layer), cotton towel, or large paper
>   coffee filters

Line a sieve or colander with a paper filter, double-layer cheesecloth, or cotton towel. Set it over a large deep bowl, pot, jar, or drip coffee maker. Pour yogurt into lined colander, cover and refrigerate 3 to 18 hours, depending upon consistency you want. Turn cheese out into another bowl, cover, and refrigerate. Discard whey.

Fruit Fool

This simple and delicious old English dessert dates back to Queen Elizabeth I. What could be better than puréed or crushed fruit with heavy cream? Or more easy that even a fool could make it?

English cooking authority Elizabeth David conjectures that the name comes from the old French *foulé,* meaning crushed. Usually crushed or stewed gooseberries, or other berries, were used, then swirled with heavy cream, egg whites, and custard. Our version calls for unsweetened fruit-flavored (strawberry or apricot) or unsweetened baby food fruit purées straight from the jar swirled with plain yogurt. The trick in serving this is to present it in chilled attractive saucers or glass dessert dishes.

Serves 4

Stage II

    6 cups plain yogurt

    3 cups unsweetened fruit-flavored applesauce

    or

    4 6-ounce jars unsweetened baby food fruit purée

Chill four dessert dishes or saucers. Divide the yogurt equally between the dishes and stroke it out, cover the surface of the dish or saucers. Divide the fruit purée equally between the four dishes or saucers and drop it in the center of the yogurt. Swirl the purée making a spiral pattern. Garnish with a sprig of mint or a thin slice of fresh fruit. Serve immediately.

Marinated Yogurt Cheese

Serves 4

Stage I

    1 recipe Easy Cheese

    ¼ cup olive oil

    2 cloves garlic, finely minced

    ½ teaspoon dried thyme

    ½ teaspoon dried rosemary

    1 tablespoon chopped fresh dill

Make Easy Cheese according to the directions. Divide into four rounds, shaping patties with your hands. Place in a wide, shallow bowl. In a medium mixing bowl, combine oil, garlic, thyme, rosemary, and dill. Pour oil-herb mixture over cheese. Let stand at room temperature for ½ hour, then cover and refrigerate overnight. Remove from refrigerator ½ hour before serving. Serve with crackers or crisp-breads as a sensational appetizer.

Narsai's Mother's Summer Drink or Soup

Narsai David, a California-born man of letters in the cooking world, harkens back to his youth for "a tangy drink, in which cucumber was ground with fresh dill or mint and diluted with water to the consistency of buttermilk." He recalls that served with a sandwich, it was a perfect summer lunch. This drink is refreshing with a hearty meat stew or as an everyday drink. With the addition of more yogurt, it makes delightful chilled, summer soup.

Serves 1

Stage I
    1½ cups plain yogurt, regular or nonfat
    ½ cucumber, peeled and cut into ½-inch pieces
    2 tablespoons chopped fresh mint or dill

In a blender, combine yogurt, cucumber, chopped mint or dill and enough water to dilute to desired consistency. For a summer drink, plain mineral water can be used instead of regular drinking water. For chilled soup, add very little water and place in refrigerator for at least 15 minutes after blending.

Chapter Nine

❧

Vegetables and Tofu

MOTHER WAS RIGHT—eat your vegetables. They are delicious over fish and rice, with or in cornmeal, grilled or roasted with chicken, steamed with ginger and garlic and, of course, with butter and salt.

Some of our favorite combinations are: carrots with fresh dill, carrots with parsnips mashed together with butter and salt, Brussels sprouts steamed with lemon and topped with butter, canned unsweetened whole corn with lime juice, Swiss chard with red onion, olive oil, and garlic, stemmed parsley with melted butter and nuts, squashes or yams with butter and salt, and baked yam with almond butter on top (a delectable breakfast).

Carrot and Leek Side Dish
Dayna's Stand-By-Dinner
Marion Cunningham's Winter Vegetable Cobbler
Old Fashioned Baked Potato Dinner
Rosie's Versatile Vegetable Ragoût
Tofu Steaks and Brown Rice

Carrot and Leek Side Dish

The delicious flavor of this colorful vegetable mixture complements the rest of any meal.

Serves 2 to 4

eek
carrots
¼ teaspoon salt
½ cup water

Wash leek and cut away and discard most of green portion. Slice white portion into ¼-inch pieces and place in medium saucepan with salt. Peel carrots, cut into ⅛-inch slices, and add to leeks. Add water to vegetables, cover, bring to a boil, then simmer for 10 to 12 minutes, until tender. Drain and serve.

Dayna's Stand-By Dinner

An efficient friend concocted this dish to ease herself into a cozy evening at home after a hectic day. Lemon juice and salt make this dish a sturdy supper with a surprisingly satisfying flavor.

Serves 1

Stage I
    olive oil for the pan
    1 yellow onion, chopped
    3 cloves garlic, chopped coarsely
    3 small boiling potatoes, sliced ¼-inch thick
    1 tablespoon fresh lemon juice
    1 8-ounce package frozen whole leaf spinach, washed and
       rough cut
    salt and pepper to taste
    1 tablespoon fresh lemon juice

Coat a heavy frying pan with enough oil to cover the bottom or spray pan with oil before heating. Heat pan over medium heat. Add onion and garlic and sauté briefly. Add potatoes, cover and cook over medium heat for 5 minutes or until the fork easily pierces potatoes. Lay spinach on top of potatoes. Cover pan for 2 to 3 minutes to allow spinach to wilt. Remove cover, drizzle lemon juice over all, add salt and pepper, and serve.

Marion Cunningham's Winter Vegetable Cobbler

Marion Cunningham's cobbler is cozy, homey, and all-American—just right for lunch with friends, and as friendly as Marion herself. If a friend asks what she can prepare for an upcoming party, hand her this recipe. Everyone will be happy!

Serves 6

    1 turnip, peeled and cut into bite-size pieces
    1 potato (russet or baking), peeled and diced
    1 celery root, peeled and diced (about 1½ cups)
    1 onion, coarsely chopped
    3 carrots, peeled and sliced
    ½ cup chopped parsley
    1 cup canned vegetable broth, chilled
    2 tablespoons cornstarch
    1 teaspoon salt
    freshly ground pepper
    2 tablespoons of butter

Cobbler dough
    1¾ cups whole-wheat pastry flour
    1 tablespoon baking powder
    ½ teaspoon salt
    6 tablespoons butter, chilled in small pieces
    ¾ cup cream

Preheat oven to 350 degrees. Put the turnip, potato, celery root, onion, carrots, and parsley in a 2 inch-deep 8-cup ovenproof baking dish. In a small mixing bowl, blend the broth with the cornstarch until smooth, pour over the vegetables, and mix well. Add salt and pepper to taste, and mix to blend. Dot the top of the vegetables with butter.

Make the cobbler dough:
In a large mixing bowl, mix flour, baking powder, and salt with a fork to blend. Drop pieces of chilled butter into flour mixture and rub quickly with fingertips until the mixture resembles bread crumbs.

Using the fork, slowly stir in the cream until roughly mixed. Gather the dough and knead five or six times. Roll out the dough on a lightly floured work surface to the size of the top of the baking dish. The dough should be about ¼ inch thick. Place the dough on top of the vegetables. Bake for 45 to 55 minutes, until vegetables are cooked through and crust is browned. Test vegetables for doneness with a knife tip.

Old Fashioned Baked Potato Dinner

With a few additions, the simple baked potato is probably the best all-around comfort food. Narsai's Versatile Savory Sauce (page 99) makes a wonderful topping.

Serves 1

Stage I
  1 large baking potato
  1 to 2 tablespoons butter or oil, to taste
  2 sardines, packed in water or oil, flaked
  and/or
  ½ cup broccoli flowerets
  salt and pepper to taste

Preheat oven to 400 degrees. Thoroughly wash potato and prick several times with a fork. Bake in oven unwrapped on rack for 40 minutes to 1 hour, or until done. Remove potato from oven and cut open. Add the butter or oil, sardines, broccoli, and salt and pepper to taste. Wrap potato in foil and return to oven for 10 minutes to let flavors meld.

Rosie's Versatile Vegetable Ragoût

Rosemary Manell, Julia Child's colleague, devised this attractive and simple dish for a tasty lunch or supper. The ragoût can be served with any whole grain noodles, brown rice, rice cakes, tortilla chips, crispbreads, or use Teff or Whole Wheat Bread(pages 88, 90). A dollop of yogurt on the side makes this dish extra special.

Serves 4 to 6

Stage I

    2 or 3 large peeled garlic cloves, cut lengthwise into slices

    1 red onion (about 8 ounces), sliced in ⅜-inch strips

    1 medium eggplant (1¼ pounds) cut into 1-inch cubes

    ½ teaspoon lemon juice

    3 bell peppers (one each of red, green, and yellow) cut in
      ⅜-inch strips

    1 tablespoon lemon juice

    1 teaspoon salt

    dash of pepper

    3 tablespoons olive oil

Stage II

    Add 1 medium diced tomato with eggplant.

Stage III

    Add ½ cup sliced mushrooms and 1 medium diced
    tomato with eggplant.

Place steamer basket in a large saucepan filled with 1½ inches boiling water. Put garlic and onion in the steamer basket, cover, and steam for 2 minutes. In a large mixing bowl, toss eggplant with lemon juice, add to steamer, cover, and steam for 3 more minutes. When tender, add peppers, cover, and steam for another 3 minutes. Test for doneness with a knife. If vegetables are not tender, add more water to the pot, cover, and steam for a few more minutes. Remove basket and let vegetables drain. Turn into a large mixing bowl and gently mix with lemon juice, salt, some freshly ground black pepper, and olive oil. Serve warm.

Tofu Steaks and Brown Rice

Tofu is made from soybeans and is one of the best, least fatty, and most inexpensive sources of protein. Here the tofu is cooked in a tasty mixture of garlic, olive oil, and soy sauce. If you have a choice at the market between the silky smooth tofu or the regular coarse variety, choose the regular. The little irregular holes allow the marinade to soak into the tofu—essential for good flavor.

Serves 2

Stage II

    2½ cups water
    ½ teaspoon salt
    ½ teaspoon butter or oil
    1 cup brown rice
    8 ounces regular tofu
    4 tablespoons olive oil
    1 teaspoon minced garlic
    3 teaspoons unsweetened, low salt soy sauce
    Optional: a few radishes, small celery stalk, small bunch
        watercress, or water chestnuts

Stage III

    Add ½ cup sliced fresh or sautéed mushrooms.

In a medium saucepan combine the water, salt, and butter or oil. When the water comes to a full boil, slowly add the brown rice. Continue to boil for a few minutes, cover, and reduce heat to simmer. The rice will take about 40 minutes to cook. After about 20 minutes, prepare the rest of the meal. Drain the tofu, cut into ½-inch thick slices, and place on paper towel to dry. Heat olive oil in a heavy skillet over medium heat. Add the garlic and soy sauce and stir. Add the tofu slices and cook gently, turning the slices over occasionally. The tofu can cook from 10 to 20 minutes and will turn a nutty brown. Wash and slice the radishes and celery. Wash and cut the watercress or other greens. When the rice is done, spoon steaming mounds onto each plate, add the tofu, and pour any remaining juices on top. Sprinkle with radishes, celery, and greens. Toasted walnuts are a delicious addition.

Chapter Ten

❧

Early Morning and Eggs

E'VE TRIED TO keep you from thinking in the old pattern of breakfast, lunch, and dinner, but for those who cling to a bowl of cereal in the early morning, here is a wholesome collection of tasty grains. Some of these recipes are adaptations from suggestions shared while standing in line at the grocery store, but mostly they are from support groups. More adventurous breakfasters are invited to look at the Scandinavian Breakfast on page 125.

As we used to say in the first grade "Mister Egg is my friend!" An egg will satisfy and sustain you at breakfast, lunch, and dinner. Try these unusual combinations. If you keep the ingredients on hand for all of these dishes, you may even try the ones you think you won't like. For a little pick me up, try a slice of either Teff or Whole Wheat Bread with a plain egg cooked your favorite way. There is really nothing better than a fresh egg with a little salt and some bread and butter.

Early Morning
Breakfast Popcorn
Charles Shere's Bog Man Cereal
Night-Before Oatmeal
Puffed Grain Cereal with Nuts

Eggs
Oven-Coddled Eggs
Scandinavian Breakfast
Scrambled or Omelet-Style Eggs
Siesta Breakfast

Breakfast Popcorn

Though popcorn isn't a usual breakfast food, it's warm, filling, hearty, and sustaining. Throw convention to the wind! Popcorn and a strong cup of Ginger Tea (page 98) make a perky combination.

Serves 1

Stage I
    1½ tablespoons olive oil
    1 teaspoon butter
    ¼ cup plain popcorn (organic)
    butter and salt to taste (optional)

Put olive oil and butter into a heavy 2-quart pot (with lid) over medium-high heat and toss in a kernel of corn. When it pops, add the rest of the popcorn, cover the pot and lower heat. Keeping the lid on tightly, move pot back and forth continuously, until popping stops. Transfer popcorn to bowl and add a little melted butter and salt, if desired.

Charles Shere's Bog Man Cereal

Charles, a member of the Chez Panisse team, devised this cereal. It was inspired by the famous Bog Man of Denmark, circa 100 A.D., who was found perfectly preserved in a peat bog with his stomach full of whole grains. If you are used to digesting and eating whole grains this cereal is a real treat! This hearty cereal breaks down slowly in the body — it will easily see you through to noon. A trip to the health food store is required, but it's worth it.

Serves 2

Stage I
>   ¼ cup each of soft white wheat kernels, red (hard) winter
>   wheat berries, rye berries, oat berries
>   ½ teaspoon salt
>   optional: Almond Milk (page 96), plain yogurt, butter,
>   olive oil

Place the grains in a medium saucepan with salt and cover with water, so that the cereal is about one-half inch below the surface. Bring to a boil, and continue to boil uncovered for about 20 minutes. Remove from heat, cover, and refrigerate overnight. In the morning, bring to a boil again and then simmer for another 20 minutes. Serve either with Almond Milk, plain yogurt, butter, or even a tablespoon of olive oil.

Night-Before Oatmeal

This marvelously nutty and extremely sustaining oatmeal offers you a healthy way to start the day.
>   Serves 1

Stage I
>   2 cups cold water
>   ½ teaspoon salt
>   ½ cup steel-cut, Irish or Scotch oats
>   Almond Milk (page 96)
>   butter to taste

Fill the bottom half of a double boiler two-thirds full of water and bring to a simmer. Process ¼ cup of oats at a time for 3 seconds in a blender. The partially chopped grain will not be uniform, giving this oatmeal a pleasing texture. Combine 2 cups cold water, salt, and oats in top half of the double boiler and bring to a boil over direct heat for a minute, then place pot over simmering water in bottom half of double boiler. Cook uncovered and stir occasionally for 45 minutes. Cover and store overnight in the refrigerator. Warm the oatmeal the next morning over low heat, adding a little water for desired consistency. Serve in a warmed bowl with Almond Milk or butter.

Puffed Grain Cereal with Nuts

This is a progressive recipe. In Stage I, use only the first three ingredients. But be of good cheer—this is tasty and toasty! As you progress, you can make additions as indicated.

Serves 1

Stage I

    1 cup of puffed whole brown rice or wheat cereal

    2 tablespoons whole almonds

    1 tablespoon Ginger Tea (page 98), Almond Milk (page 96) or hot water

Stage II

    the above, plus ½ peach or apple, cut into small pieces

    1 tablespoon milk

Stage III

    All of the above, plus 1 apple, grated, or small pieces of pear, plum, and a few grapes

    1 tablespoon heavy cream

Preheat oven to 375 degrees. Pour puffed rice and almonds on separate baking sheets, place in oven, and bake for 10 minutes. With rolling pin, roughly crush the toasted almonds on baking sheet. Place rice and nuts in a bowl, add fruit when appropriate for each stage. Sprinkle with the appropriate liquids above.

Oven-Coddled Eggs

This simple recipe gives you a nicely textured "soft-boiled" egg. Your oven does all the work.

Serves 1

Stage I

Preheat oven to 275 degrees. Put whole egg (in shell) in a muffin tin or on foil and place in oven for 15 minutes. Turn finished egg out onto dish or eat out of shell. Season with salt and pepper.

Scandinavian Breakfast

If sardines had another name, I'm sure everyone would eat these delightful silvery little protein packets more frequently. A few at breakfast with an egg and you'll sail through to lunch. This combination is particularly popular in Norway.

Serves 1

Stage I
    oil for the pan
    2 eggs
    2 rice cakes or crispbread
    one-half tin (3¾-ounce size) good quality sardines packed
       in oil or water
    1 tablespoon chopped fresh chives
    butter as desired
    salt to taste

Warm plate in 200 degree oven. Lightly oil a medium-sized pan. Beat eggs lightly and scramble in pan. While the eggs are cooking, lightly toast rice cakes in oven (watch carefully to keep from burning). Remove warm plate from oven. Place eggs, sardines, chives, and rice cakes in a circle on warmed plate. Add butter and salt as desired.

Scrambled or Omelet-Style Eggs

Nothing makes a more flexible meal than scrambled eggs. They're uncomplicated (it was the only thing Eleanor Roosevelt knew how to make) and you'll find many suggestions below to include in the eggs or place on top.

Serves 2

Stage I
    4 eggs
    1 teaspoon olive oil
    ½ cup toasted chopped almonds

or

½ cup cooked wild rice or brown rice/wild rice
combination

or

½ cup toasted, broken tortilla chips, crackers, matzos, rice
cakes, chopped fresh herbs, or pieces of red or green
bell pepper

Stage II

½ cup cottage cheese, ricotta cheese, or salsa without
sweetener

In a small mixing bowl, break the eggs and stir together with a
fork until yolk and white are well mixed. Heat a heavy skillet to
medium heat. Add enough olive oil to coat bottom of pan, add eggs
and preferred additions. Stir mixture quickly until eggs are cooked.
Turn out onto plates with a spatula and serve.

Siesta Breakfast

This combination of cooked beans and eggs is common almost anywhere "south of the border." It's a very warm and comforting breakfast welcome by anyone.

Serves 1

Stage I

1 egg
1 cup cooked beans (garbanzo, lima, black-eyed peas,
kidney)
salt and pepper to taste
1 tablespoon unsweetened salsa
½ tablespoon chopped fresh herbs
1 teaspoon toasted nuts

Preheat oven to 275 degrees. Put whole egg (in shell) in a muffin tin or on foil and place in oven for 15 minutes. Purée cooked
beans and some of their liquid for 5 seconds in blender. Consistency

Early Morning and Eggs

should be chunky, not soupy. Add salt and pepper, if desired. Scoop onto heat-proof dish. When timer sounds, turn off oven, remove egg and set aside and put dish of beans in oven. Make toast and tea (about 7–10 minutes). Remove beans from oven, scoop egg out of shell over them or to the side. Season as desired with additional salt and pepper, unsweetened salsa, chopped fresh herbs, and toasted nuts.

127

Chapter Eleven

❧

Rice, Cornmeal, and Pasta

ROWN RICE IS a staple in many households and during your recovery we hope it will be one of yours. Here's a collection of suggestions for cooking with brown rice. These recipes are also good for basmati, or any rice you prefer.

Cornmeal can sustain you throughout the day—ask any American homesteader. Undegerminated cornmeal, another way of saying whole cornmeal, is also called whole corn cereal, cornmeal mush, or polenta. It's good any way you eat it. It is especially important to try to buy undegerminated (whole) cornmeal for Stage I. There are many different grain sizes of cornmeal; the smaller grains will cook more quickly. The minimum cooking time will be about three to five minutes depending on the size of the grains.

Any time you make pasta, it is open season on leftovers. Feel free to experiment and add your own ideas to the recipes. For variety, try different kinds of noodles, especially rice flour and Japanese buckwheat noodles.

Rice
Basic Brown Rice
Brown Rice and Toasted Nuts with Creamy Polenta
Pilaf

Cornmeal
Hot Corn Cereal
Polenta

Pasta
Rosie's Posie Pasta
Seated Garlic Pasta

Basic Brown Rice

Brown rice is one of the best foods for your body. The variations can turn it into a quick, nutritious, and satisfying meal. Carrots and leeks make a particularly tasty combination. This recipe is also good for basmati rice.

Serves 4

Stage I
2½ cups boiling water
1 cup raw brown rice
1 teaspoon salt

In a medium saucepan, boil the water. Add rice and salt, stir, and briefly bring to a boil. Reduce to simmer, cover, and cook for 45 minutes.

Variations
Wash and cut one leek into ⅛ inch rounds, discarding most of green part. Cut one carrot like the leek and coarsely chop a small bunch of parsley. Add vegetables to rice before covering saucepan. Serve with a dollop of plain yogurt.

Preheat oven to 250 degrees. Place ½ cup shelled almonds on a baking sheet and roast for 20 minutes. Remove when lightly brown and set aside. (For more flavor, nuts can be crushed or chopped.) Wash and stem ½ bunch of watercress. Serve rice topped with nuts and watercress on the side.

Brown Rice and Toasted Nuts with Creamy Polenta

Have two staples ready before you build this intriguing little dish: cooked brown rice and toasted almond or cashew pieces. The cornmeal cooks quickly and is poured over the top. Nuts are added, then the dish is garnished with radishes or any crunchy and colorful vegetable.

Serves 1

Stage I
>   1 cup cooked brown rice
>   ⅓ cup undegerminated cornmeal
>   1 cup boiling water
>   dash of salt
>   1 tablespoon butter (optional)
>   ½ cup toasted almond or cashew pieces
>   2 radishes, thinly sliced

Warm plate in a 200 degree oven. Heat the cooked brown rice in a medium saucepan with a bit of water over medium heat. In a separate pan, add cornmeal to boiling water and salt. Whisk over medium heat without stopping until lumps disappear and cornmeal is smooth and pourable. Add more water if necessary and butter, if desired. Remove plate from oven. Place brown rice on plate, pour cornmeal over rice, add nuts, and garnish with radishes.

Pilaf

Sharon Cadwallader is well-known syndicated food writer. Her wonderful idea about how to prepare brown rice before you cook it makes this an especially delicious pilaf.

Serves 3

Stage I
>   1 cup brown rice
>   2 tablespoons butter
>   ½ cup chopped onion
>   1 cup chopped carrots

1 clove minced garlic
2 chopped scallions
2½ cups chicken broth
½ teaspoon salt
¼ cup toasted pine nuts or almonds
3 tablespoons parsley, chopped

Preheat oven to 350 degrees. Place rice in baking pan and bake for 15 minutes. In a skillet on medium heat, melt butter, add onion, carrots, garlic, and scallions and sauté until onions are transparent. Add the oven-dried rice, broth, and salt to vegetable mixture. Stir once, bring to a boil, reduce heat, and cover. Cook for 35 to 40 minutes, or until vegetables are tender. Add nuts and parsley, toss lightly and serve.

Hot Corn Cereal

This takes only three or four minutes to put together. Corn is extremely nourishing and sustaining. Best of all, it will sustain you until noon or perhaps even dinner time. In the frontier days, this dish might have been called Company Cornmeal Mush.

Serves 1

Stage I
1¼ cups water
⅓ cup undegerminated cornmeal
¼ teaspoon salt
butter (optional)

In a medium saucepan, bring water to boil. Add cornmeal slowly to water and whisk without stopping until lumps disappear. Add salt. Or whisk together water, cornmeal, and salt and bring to a boil, whisking or stirring occasionally. When the cornmeal begins to pull away from the sides of the saucepan, remove from heat. Pour into a warmed cereal bowl, top with butter and enjoy.

Polenta

This recipe is one of the simplest and tastiest hot meals you can make for yourself.

Serves 1

Stage I

    2 cups boiling water
    ¾ cup undegerminated cornmeal
    ¼ teaspoon salt
    ¼ cup broccoli florets
    2 cloves minced garlic
    small pinch fresh rosemary
    butter to taste

Stage II

Add one medium chopped or 4 cut cherry tomatoes, or 2 tablespoons unsweetened salsa to cooked polenta before serving.

In a medium saucepan, bring water to boil. Add cornmeal slowly to water and whisk without stopping until lumps disappear. Add salt, broccoli, garlic, and rosemary. When the cornmeal begins to pull away from the sides of the saucepan, remove from heat. Dot with butter and eat immediately.

Rosie's Posie Pasta

In this inspired recipe by Rosemary Manell, Julia Child's long-time cooking colleague, dollops of piquant salsa are placed at the edge of the pasta, making a bright ring of red roses. It's pretty and truly delicious. Ms. Manell once served this elegant lunch with three perfect enormous succulent strawberries. Only a superlative cook can pull that off! In Stage III, add a little freshly grated Parmesan cheese.

Serves 1

Stage II

    1 quart water
    2 ounces spaghetti noodles

2 chopped cloves garlic
salt to taste
1 cup broccoli florets
2 tablespoons salsa without sweeteners
olive oil

Stage III
Add 1 tablespoon freshly grated Parmesan cheese.

In a large pot, bring water to a boil. Break pasta in half and add to pot with garlic. When water returns to boil, add salt. Cook pasta until *al dente,* not more than 15 minutes. Remove from heat and pour into a colander over a large bowl to drain, saving the hot water. To warm a serving bowl, pour in 1 cup of the hot water. Pour the remaining water back into the pot and bring to a boil. Add broccoli, cook for a couple minutes until tender-crisp, then drain. Discard water from serving bowl. Coat bowl lightly with olive oil, turn in spaghetti, add broccoli, and toss with a bit more oil.

Dot rosettes of salsa around the edge of the pasta. Serve immediately while hot, or even later at room temperature.

Variation
Cut green cabbage or fennel (or a combination of both) into ⅓-inch slices, enough for 1 cup. Boil for 30 seconds and combine with pasta.

Seated Garlic Pasta

Standing up to peel garlic can be tiring. Pull up a stool and sit down. This pasta is sure to become a favorite tasty, light meal.

Serves 2

Stage I
6 to 8 cloves garlic
1 teaspoon salt
4 ounces whole grain pasta noodles
2 quarts water

olive oil or spray for the pan
butter or olive oil to taste

Separate and peel garlic cloves, drop into boiling water in a saucepan for 30 seconds, remove with a slotted spoon, and drain. In a large pot, add salt and pasta to boiling water; keep at rolling boil for 8 to 13 minutes. Cook pasta until *al dente,* not more than 15 minutes. While pasta is boiling, sauté garlic cloves in heated olive oil in heavy frying pan, turning as needed until the cloves become pecan colored (they must not get dark or they will be bitter). Drain pasta, add to garlic in frying pan, and mix thoroughly. Add salt and butter or olive oil to taste and serve on a warm plate.

Chapter Twelve

Chicken and Seafood

C HICKEN IS EVERYBODY'S favorite standby dinner. It's important that you try to get the best-tasting chicken you can— one that is fresh and range-fed. Our favorite recipe in this section is Chicken with Roasted Red Peppers. This dish was a hit with Helen's family during her bout with Candida and has remained a favorite ever since.

Always try to buy fresh fish from *a trusted source*—not always easy, but worth the effort. If your choice is between long-frozen fish and canned fish, choose canned. It's actually safer for the Candida patient and is tastier. A piece of good fish rolled in Teff (page 88) or Whole Wheat (page 90) bread crumbs, seasoned, pan-fried in olive oil and butter, and served with lots of lemon and steamed vegetables makes a perfect lunch or dinner with hardly any fuss.

Chicken
Chicken with Roasted Red Peppers
Company Chicken Dinner with Yogurt-Lemon Sauce
Helen's Versatile Party Chicken
Narsai David's Chicken Stew

Seafood
Basic Tuna Sandwich
Pan-Fried Crunchy Catfish and Golden Crookneck Squash

Peel and Eat Shrimp
Salmon Patties
Wolfgang Puck's Bay Scallops with Sautéed Apples

Chicken with Roasted Red Peppers

This recipe was created because there was nothing left in the refrigerator but chicken pieces and one jar of roasted red bell peppers. What a lovely dish it created! I browned the chicken, emptied the contents of the bottle over the chicken pieces, turned on the oven and forgot about it. Forty-five minutes later my family and I had a wonderful dinner. Polenta (page 133) is a perfect accompaniment.
Serves 4

Stage I
    oil for the pan
    1 whole chicken cut into small pieces or 2 whole chicken breasts, quartered, trimmed of extra skin (8 pieces)
    2 7-ounce jars roasted red bell peppers

Preheat oven to 375 degrees. In a heavy frying pan, heat enough oil to cover the bottom, or spray pan with oil before heating over medium-high heat. Lightly brown the chicken pieces on all sides. Pour the peppers and juices over the chicken. Cover pan, transfer to the oven, and bake for 45 minutes.

Company Chicken Dinner with Yogurt-Lemon Sauce

This recipe is a simple way to make a meal for friends while you rest.
Serves 4

Stage I
    4 chicken breast halves
    4 cloves garlic, cut in half
    1 cup plain yogurt
    juice of 1 lemon
    2 10-ounce packages frozen baby peas

butter

1 tablespoon chopped fresh herb (basil, tarragon, or oregano)

Stage II

Add 2 teaspoons whole mustard seed on dollop of yogurt.

Preheat oven to 350 degrees. Arrange chicken breasts skin side up on a baking sheet with sides. Place two garlic clove halves on each breast. Combine yogurt with lemon juice. (In Stage II, you can also add mustard seed.) Spoon a large dollop on top of each breast. Bake for approximately one hour. Shortly before chicken is ready, cook peas for two minutes in a little less water than package directs. Serve chicken and peas on warm plates, topping peas with a bit of butter and fresh herb.

Helen's Versatile Party Chicken

With very little effort, you can do so much with this recipe. By adding chicken broth and almond butter, along with vegetables and cooked brown rice, it makes a delightful soup.

Serves 6

Stage I

1 whole 4 pound chicken, trimmed of fat, wings, and extra skin

oil for the pan

1½ teaspoons chopped fresh basil

¾ teaspoon chopped fresh oregano

½ teaspoon salt

½ teaspoon pepper

2 chopped cloves garlic

4 carrots

3 red potatoes

1 small onion (optional)

2 stalks celery (optional)

1 lemon, halved

Preheat oven to 350 degrees. In a heavy frying pan, heat enough oil to cover the bottom, or spray pan with oil before heating over medium-high heat. Place whole chicken in the pan and brown on one side for about 5 minutes. Turn and brown the other side. Turn chicken on its back, sprinkle with herbs and seasonings, and continue browning. Chop garlic, cut carrots, potatoes, onion, and celery into one-inch chunks. Add chopped vegetables to pan, cover, and put in the oven for 1¼ hours. Squeeze lemon over the chicken. Carve and serve with vegetables.

Variation

Prepare chicken as above. Strip carcass of meat and cut into bite-sized chunks. In a large pot, add 4 cups of chicken broth, 2 cups of cooked brown rice, and the chicken. Add almond butter to desired thickness. Cover and simmer on low-medium heat for 20 minutes or until vegetables are cooked through.

Narsai David's Chicken Stew

When you long for a warm, comforting stew, this will fill the bill. A little bit of this, a little bit of that, put it all in a little pan and you have dinner. Either Teff or Whole Wheat Bread (page 88, 90) is a delicious complement.

Serves 1

Stage I
> 2 small chicken backs or thighs, cut into pieces
> ¼ teaspoon salt
> ½ carrot
> ½ stalk celery
> ½ onion
> ½ potato
> 2 sprigs parsley
> 1 clove garlic
> 2 whole peppercorns
> 1 bay leaf

2 whole cloves
1½ cups chicken broth

Trim the chicken of any excess skin, or remove skin altogether. Place chicken in a medium-sized pot and season with salt. Cut carrot, celery, onion, and potato into small pieces and add to the pot. Pinch the leaves off a sprig or two of parsley and put them in. Peel garlic, cut in half, and add to the pot along with peppercorns and bay leaf stuck with cloves. Pour in chicken broth to barely cover chicken pieces. Heat and bring to boil, then cover and reduce heat to gentle simmer for 30 minutes. Remove bay leaf and cloves with a slotted spoon. Adjust seasoning if necessary. Serve with Teff or Whole Wheat Bread.

Basic Tuna Sandwich

A decent tuna fish salad sandwich on whole wheat is an American birthright. But for the Candida dieter, mayonnaise has been the difficulty. Here's a delicious and healthy solution. Serve with Teff or Whole Wheat Bread (page 88, 90).

Makes 3 sandwiches

Stage I
    1 6½-ounce can water packed tuna
    ¾ cup plain yogurt
    salt and pepper, to taste
    lemon juice, to taste
    chopped fresh dill (optional)

Drain the water from tuna, place in mixing bowl, and flake with a fork. Add other ingredients to bowl and mix well. Spread on crisp bread, crackers, Teff or Whole Wheat Bread.

Variation
Stuff tuna mixture into red or green bell pepper and eat as cold salad.

Pan-Fried Crunchy Catfish
and Golden Crookneck Squash

Your plate will take on a yummy golden hue with this combination.

Serves 1

Stage I

    ½ cup undegerminated cornmeal

    freshly ground black pepper to taste

    oil for the pan

    1 catfish fillet (¾ to 1 inch thick)

    1 clove garlic, sliced

    3 small yellow crookneck squash, cut into ¼-inch thick
        slices

    1 lemon

    2 sprigs parsley

In a shallow dish mix together cornmeal and dash of freshly ground black pepper. In a heavy frying pan, heat enough oil to cover the bottom, or spray pan with oil before heating over medium heat. Dredge catfish in cornmeal mixture and add to hot frying pan. When fish is golden brown on one side, turn it, push it to the side of the pan, and add garlic and squash. Toss the vegetables with a spatula as they cook and brown. Sprinkle juice from half of the lemon over all when fish is cooked. Serve with lemon slices and parsley sprigs for garnish.

Peel and Eat Shrimp

High in protein and easy to prepare, this dish offers good eating at any time of the day.

Serves 1

Stage I

    6 large unpeeled shrimp or prawns

    1 cup boiling water

    lettuce and/or parsley

lemon juice
freshly ground black pepper
rye crackers

Toss shrimp into enough boiling water to cover. Remove the shrimp when they turn pink (about 5 minutes), drain, and set aside. Arrange lettuce and/or parsley on a serving plate. Shell the shrimp and arrange on the bed of lettuce and/or parsley. Drizzle shrimp with lemon juice, and grind fresh black pepper over all. Serve with rye crackers—delicious!

Salmon Patties

A megadose of exciting fresh green cilantro brings new spirit to this old favorite, which is good at all stages of the diet. Try the patties with Carrot and Leek Side Dish (page 115) for a well-balanced treat. Leftover patties can be frozen.

Serves 3

Stage I
    1 8-ounce can of pink salmon, slightly drained
    1 clove garlic, minced
    ½ teaspoon salt
    1 egg, beaten
    1 cup chopped cilantro
    1 cup (about 6) crushed crispbread crackers
    oil for the pan
    lemon juice to taste

Mix the salmon, garlic, and salt with beaten egg. Add chopped cilantro and crushed crackers and continue to mix until well-combined. Pat mixture into three hamburger-size patties about ⅓-inch thick. In a heavy frying pan, heat enough oil to cover the bottom or spray pan with oil before heating over medium-high heat. Sauté patties briefly on both sides, about 2 minutes each side.

Squeeze lemon juice over the patties to taste.

Wolfgang Puck's Bay Scallops with Sautéed Apples

A surprising and elegant combination—perfect for a small dinner party in Stage II.

Serves 6

Stage II
- 2 pippin or Granny Smith apples
- 2 tablespoons unsalted butter
- 1 pound fresh baby bay scallops
- salt to taste
- freshly ground white pepper, to taste
- 1 tablespoon almond or safflower oil
- 1 tablespoon chopped fresh Italian parsley or cilantro

Peel, halve, and core the apples. Slice them thinly or cut them into ¼-inch julienne strips. Heat a large frying pan and add the butter. Sauté the apples over moderate heat 2 to 3 minutes, or until they are slightly brown but still crispy. Sauté the apples (and scallops) in several small batches instead of crowding your pan. Season the scallops with salt and pepper. Heat another large frying pan and add oil. Sauté the scallops over high heat until just springy to the touch, from 30 seconds to 1 minute, depending on their size. Remove from heat. Stir parsley into scallops and correct seasoning. Arrange the apple slices in a wreath on warm appetizer plates and place the scallops in the center of the wreaths. Garnish with sprigs of Italian parsley or cilantro.

Chapter Thirteen

※

Julia Child's Special Dinner

H ELEN WAS INTRODUCED to Julia Child through food world connections. At a Chez Panisse lunch, Helen described the work in progress on this book and Ms. Child generously offered to contribute not just a recipe but an entire menu. We have reproduced her recipes exactly as she sent them to us. Her instructions are as friendly and helpful as the dishes are elegant and delicious. You need not feel left out when you can invite guests to a special dinner designed for you by Julia Child herself!

Menu
Poached Fish Steaks with Lemon Butter Sauce and Garlic
     Mashed Potatoes or
Braised Celery or Celery Victor (Stage I)
Celery Remoulade (Stage II)

Poached Fish Steaks with Lemon Butter Sauce

An easy and delightful way to prepare fish steaks such as salmon, cod, or halibut, are to poach them in a pan of lightly salted water flavored with lemon. They take eight to ten minutes to cook and can wait in their cooking liquid for fifteen to twenty minutes before serving. For dieters, serve the fish simply with lemon wedges, and for others you can pass melted butter or a lemon butter sauce.
     Serves 6

6 fish steaks, 8 ounces each and about ¾ inch thick, kept
    in ice until you are ready to cook them
1 or 2 wide saucepans with 4 inches of boiling water
2 teaspoons of salt and 2 tablespoons of lemon juice per
    quart of water

For lemon butter sauce:
3 tablespoons (about ¾ cup) lemon juice
¼ teaspoon salt
white pepper to taste
1½ sticks chilled unsalted butter cut into 16 to 18 pieces
minced fresh herbs such as parsley, dill, or chives
    (optional)

Poaching the fish

Fifteen to twenty minutes before you plan to serve, set out your
fish, have the water at the boil, and add the salt and lemon juice.
One by one, lay the fish steaks in the water, and maintain it at the
almost simmer—no real bubbles, but a shivering movement in the
water. Set timer for 8 minutes, and when the time is up, turn off the
heat but let the fish rest in water for 2 minutes—or a few minutes
longer if you are not ready to serve.

The lemon butter sauce

While the fish steaks are poaching, bring the lemon juice to the
boil in a small stainless saucepan with ¼ teaspoon of salt and several grinds of white pepper, letting liquid boil down and reduce
almost to a glaze in the pan, to about one tablespoon. Then, a piece
or two at a time, and holding the pan at the side of the heat, start
beating in the butter with a wire whisk, adding another piece as
each addition has almost absorbed. The chilled butter creams and
remains butter-colored rather than clear like melted butter, and the
sauce should be creamy, almost like a hollandaise. When all the butter has gone in, taste and correct seasoning. Keep pan near the fish-
poaching pan, so that it will stay tepid but not warm—or the butter
will thin out and lose its creamy quality. Whisk in the optional herbs.

Serving

When the fish is done and you are ready to serve, dip it out with a slotted spatula and drain on a clean folded towel before placing on a hot platter or plates. Spoon a bit of sauce over each serving, and accompany with boiled new potatoes, sauteed cucumbers, fresh peas or asparagus tips, or a combination of sliced cucumbers and tomatoes with watercress. Pass a dish of lemon wedges along with the sauce.

Braised Garlic

Garlic loses its fiery bite when thoroughly cooked, but retains its wonderful flavor.

Stage I
    2 or 3 heads of large garlic cloves (or elephant garlic that you may wish to halve or quarter)
    2 tablespoons butter
    ½ cup beef or chicken stock

Special equipment suggested: small heavy-bottomed covered saucepan.

Braising the garlic

Separate the garlic cloves and drop them into a pan of boiling water for thirty seconds. Drain, and slip off the skins. Heat the butter in the saucepan and sauté the garlic cloves slowly for two minutes without coloring it. Add the stock, cover, and simmer slowly 20 to 30 minutes until tender but the garlic holds its shape. Set aside. Add to beef or chicken stew, braised vegetables, or to mashed potatoes as in the following suggestion.

Garlic Mashed Potatoes

Serves 6

Stage I
    1 recipe Braised Garlic
    ½ cup unsalted beef or chicken stock

salt to taste

5 to 6 cups homemade mashed potatoes

When the Braised Garlic has simmered and is tender, add the stock and a little salt to taste. Simmer 5 to 10 minutes longer, until garlic is very tender and easily mashed. Add the garlic to the potatoes as you are mashing them; season to taste and finish them as usual.

Braised Celery or Celery Victor

Celery, with its distinctive flavor and unmistakable shape, makes a fine accompaniment to roasts, steaks, hamburgers, or a vegetable plate. Cold braised celery with a decorative topping makes a perfect beginning to a meal or a companion to cold meats or a cold salad platter. Whether you are serving it hot or cold, it needs a long slow simmering with aromatic vegetables and herbs, and the following recipe is the first step.

Serves 8

Stage I

 2 large heads celery (or 3 or 4 celery hearts)

 1 large onion, sliced

 1 large carrot, sliced

 2 tablespoons olive oil or butter

 An herb packet (4 sprigs of parsley, 1 large bay leaf, and ¼ teaspoon thyme tied in washed cheesecloth)

 Liquid to come ¾ the way up the celery: chicken stock, water

 salt and pepper

While you are preparing the celery, cook the sliced onion and carrot slowly in the oil or butter in a casserole or baking dish large enough to hold the celery. Meanwhile, remove any tough stalks from the celery heads, leaving just those you judge will be tender when cooked—no tough strings to them, in other words. Cut off the tops to make the heads seven to eight inches long, or whatever the length of your casserole; trim the roots, being careful not to detach the stalks, and quarter the heads lengthwise. (Save trimmings for soups.)

When the onion and carrot are fairly tender but not browned, remove half of them from the casserole and lay in the celery, spreading the removed vegetables over the lengths of celery. Add the herb packet and liquid, and salt lightly to taste.

Bring to simmer on top of the stove, cover closely, and cook either in a 350 degree oven or on top of the stove for about 1¼ hours, basting with liquid in casserole frequently. The celery is done when it is very tender but still holds its shape. Let cool in the cooking liquid, basting frequently. (Or drape with very well washed cheesecloth, basting it well with the cooking liquid—strands of cloth will act like a wick, or an automatic baster, drawing liquid over the celery.)

To serve hot

Bring again to the simmer, basting. Remove celery to a hot platter and keep warm while rapidly boiling down the cooking liquid until it is almost syrupy. Correct seasoning and, if you wish, swirl in several tablespoons of soft butter—off heat. Spoon the liquid over the celery, sprinkle with chopped parsley, and serve.

To serve cold—*as* Celery Victor

This recipe was made famous by Chef Victor Hirtzler, of the St. Francis Hotel in San Francisco, way back in the early part of this century. As with most historic dishes, there are many versions, and this is my favorite of those I know.

Remove the braised celery to a platter, gently squeezing out excess cooking liquids; arrange it nicely in one layer, cut side up. Rapidly boil down the cooking liquid until almost syrupy. Blend ¼ cup of the liquid with one tablespoon of lemon juice; beat in one tablespoon minced shallots or scallions and whisk in, by droplets, ⅓ to ½ cup of olive oil. Season carefully with salt and pepper; then spoon over the celery; let macerate ten minutes, then tip the platter and baste celery with the sauce, repeating several times. Just before serving, make a mixture of three tablespoons chopped parsley, tossed with a little salt and pepper; strew this over the celery, and decorate with crossed strips of red pimiento and anchovies.

Celery Remoulade

That big, brown, knobby, ugly vegetable known as celery root or celeriac is almost snowy white inside, and makes a marvelous salad, or an accompaniment to smoked or boiled fish, cold cuts or other vegetables.

Manufacturing note: Celery root can be tough unless very finely shredded; you need a machine to do that for you.

Makes about one quart or serves 6 to 8

Stage II
   1 pound celery root (3 to 3½ inches across)

Tenderizing marinade:
   1½ teaspoon salt
   1½ teaspoon lemon juice

Dressing:
   ¼ cup Dijon mustard
   3 tablespoon boiling water
   ⅓ to ½ cup olive oil or salad oil
   2 tablespoons lemon juice
   salt and pepper

Optional addition:
   2 to 3 tablespoons chopped fresh parsley

Special equipment suggested: food processor with fine shredding disk, or hand-crank julienne mill; two three-quart mixing bowls, one set over a pan of simmering water.

Preparing the celery root
To prevent the celery from discoloring, work quickly. Peel the brown outside off the celery root with a short stout knife, cut into one-inch chunks, and shred in the machine. At once, toss into the cool bowl with the salt and lemon juice—lemon helps prevent dis-

coloration, and lemon and salt together have a mildly tenderizing effect. (If you are doubling or tripling the recipe, shred and season in batches.) Let steep twenty minutes.

Dressing

Meanwhile, set the warm bowl on your work surface, stir in the mustard and by dribbles whisk in the boiling water, then the oil; finally dribble and whisk in the lemon juice to make a thick creamy sauce.

Assembling

Taste the celery: if it seems salty, rinse it in cold water, drain, and dry it. Fold it into the sauce, and correct seasoning. Fold with the optional parsley.

Ahead-of-time note: The celery root is ready to serve now, but will be more tender if it is kept covered for several hours in the refrigerator—where it will keep nicely for several days.

Chapter Fourteen

The Food Directory:
An Alphabetical List of Foods

The Food Directory is an alphabetical listing of many different foods. Each food is followed by a description of the item and appropriate stage in which it can be eaten. This handy list will be helpful as a quick reference guide to any food.

A

Abalone (seafood)—Stages I, II, & III

Acidophilus (lactobacillus acidophilus and bifidus)—without sweetener in Stages I, II, & III

Acorn Squash (vegetable)—Stages I, II, & III

Adzuki Bean (legume)—see *Beans*

Agar Agar (seaweed)—fresh in Stage I; dried in Stages II & III

Aguamiel (sweetener)—when diet is completed

Albacore (seafood)—Stages I, II, & III

Alcohol (beverage—all types)—when diet is completed

Alfalfa (sprouts)—Stages I, II, & III

Alligator (meat)—Stages I, II, & III

Allspice (pimenta—spice)—Stages II & III

Almond (nut)—Stages I, II, & III

Almond Paste—when diet is completed

Aloe Vera (herb)—Stages I, II, & III

Amaranth (grain)—Stages I, II, & III

Amazake (sweetener from rice)—when diet is completed

Amberjack (seafood)—Stages I, II, & III

American Eel (seafood)—Stages I, II, & III

Anchovy (seafood)—Stages I, II, & III

Anchovy Paste (condiment)—Stages II & III, after introducing
  vinegar

Angelica (herb)—Stages II & III

Angler Fish (monkfish—seafood)—Stages I, II, & III

Anise (herb)—fresh in Stage I; dried in Stages II & III

Annatto (natural coloring)—Stages I, II, & III

Antelope (meat)—Stages I, II, & III

Apple (fruit)—Stages II & III

Apple Butter—without sweetener in Stages II & III

Apple Cider (fruit juice)—when diet is completed

Apple Cider Vinegar (vinegar)—Stages II & III

Apple Juice (drink)—when diet is completed

Apple Mint (herb)—Stages II & III

Apple Sauce—without sweetener in Stages II & III

Apricot (fruit)—Stages II & III

Arrowroot (starch)—Brazilian, Colocasia, East Indian, Fiji,
  Florida, Musa, Queenland—Stages II & III

Artichoke (vegetable)—Stages II & III

Arugula (rocket, rugula & rucola—salad greens)—Stages I, II, & III

Asafetida (asafoetida—flavoring)—Stages II & III

Asian Pear (fruit)—Stages II & III

Asparagus (vegetable)—Stages I, II, & III

Aspartame (artificial sweetener)—Stages I, II, & III; to be used in
  moderation

Atemoya (fruit)—Stages II & III

Avocado (fruit)—Stages II & III

B

Baba Ghanoush (spread or dip)—puréed eggplant, tahini (sesame
  seed butter), olive oil, lemon juice and garlic; Stages I, II, & III

Bacon (meat)—when diet is completed

Bagel (baked yeast product)—without sweetener in Stage III

Baguette (baked yeast product)—without sweetener in Stage III

Baking Powder (leavening agent)—Stages I, II, & III

Baking Soda (leavening agent)—Stages I, II, & III

Baker's Yeast (leavening agent)—see *Yeast*

Balsamic Vinegar—see *Vinegar*

Bamboo Shoots (vegetable)—Stages I, II, & III

Banana (fruit)—Stages II & III

Barbecue Sauce (condiment)—without sweetener and after introducing vinegar in Stage II & III

Barberry (fruit)—Stages II & III

Barley (grain)—whole not pearl in Stage I; pearled in II & III

Barley Malt (sweetener)—when diet is completed

Barracuda (seafood)—Stages I, II, & III

Basil (herb)—fresh in Stage I; dried in Stages II & III

Basmati Rice (grain)—brown in Stages I; white in Stages II & III

Bass—black and yellow (seafood)—Stages I, II, & III

Bay Leaf (spice)—fresh in Stage I; dried in Stages II & III

Beans (legumes—dried)—any fresh cooked without sweetener in all Stages; canned and without sweetener and tomato sauce in Stages II & III

Beans (legumes—fresh)—all types in Stages I, II, & III

Bean Curd—see *Tofu*

Bean Sprouts (germinated beans)—Stages II & III

Bear (meat)—Stages I, II, & III

Bearberry (fruit)—Stages II & III

Beef (meat)—Stages I, II, & III, preferably without hormones or steroids

Beefalo (meat)—Stages I, II, & III

Beer—see *Alcohol*

Beet (vegetable)—Stages I, II, & III

Beet Juice (vegetable juice)—Stages II & III

Beet Sugar (sweetener)—when diet is completed

Bell Pepper (sweet pepper—vegetable)—Stages I, II, & III

Bergamot (oil from a special orange)—Stages I, II, & III

Bergamont Mint (herb)—fresh in Stage I; dried in Stages II & III

Bicarbonate of Soda—see *Baking Soda*

Bilberry (whortleberry—fruit)—Stages II & III

Birds (fowl)—see individual names-all types, Stages I , II & III; preferably without antibiotics

Biscuit (baked product)—without sweetener and using appropriate grains suggested for Stages I, II, & III

Bitter Melon (fruit)—fresh in Stage III; dried when diet is completed

Blackberry (fruit)—Stages II & III

Black Beans (legume)—see *Beans*

Black-eyed peas (legume)—Stages I, II, & III

Black Pepper (seasoning)—Stages I, II, & III

Black Salsify (oyster plant-vegetable)—Stages I, II, & III

Black Walnut (nut)—see *Walnut*

Blood Orange (fruit)—Stage II & III

Blueberry (fruit)—Stages II & III

Blue Corn (grain)—Stages I, II, & III

Bluefish (seafood)—Stages I, II, & III

Bockwurst—see *Sausage*

Bok Choy (pak choi—vegetable)—Stages I, II, & III

Bologna (baloney)—see *Sandwich-Meats*

Bonito (seafood)—Stages I, II, & III

Borscht (beet soup)—without vinegar in Stage I; without sweeteners in all Stages

Boston Marrow (vegetable—squash)—Stages I, II, & III

Borage (herb)—fresh in Stage I; dried in Stages II & III

Bouillon (broth—clear soup)—freshly made in Stage I; canned, without sweetener in Stage II & III

Bow Stick (tea)—see *Pau d'Arco*

Boysenberry (fruit)—Stages II & III

Bran (Miller's bran—grain)—unprocessed in Stage I; processed in Stages II & III

Brandy (alcohol beverage)—see *Alcohol*

Brazil Nut (nut)—Stages I, II, & III
Breadfruit (fruit)—Stages II & III
Bread (baked product)—with baker's yeast, Stage III
Bread (baked product)—without baker's yeast and sweeteners
    (quick breads)—Stages I, II, & III
Brewer's Yeast (nutritional yeast)—see *Yeast*
Broccoli (vegetable)—Stages I, II, & III
Broth (bouillon—clear soup)—fresh or canned,without
    sweetener in Stages I, II, & III
Brown Rice (grain)—Stages I, II, & III
Brown Sugar (sweetener)—when diet is completed
Brussels sprout (vegetable)—Stages I, II, & III
Buckwheat (grain)—Stages I, II, & III
Buffalo (meat)—Stages I, II, & III
Bulgur (bulghur wheat—grain)—Stages I, II, & III
Burbot (seafood)—Stages I, II, & III
Burdock Root (vegetable)—Stages I, II, & III
Burnet (herb)—Stages II & III
Butter (dairy)—Stages I, II, & III
Buttermilk (dairy)—Stages II & III
Buttercup squash (vegetable)—Stages I, II, & III
Butterfish (seafood)—Stages I, II, & III
Butternut (white walnut—nut)—Stage III
Butternut Squash (vegetable)—Stages I, II, & III

C

Cabbage (vegetable)—Stages I, II, & III
Cake (confectionery)—when diet is completed
Calamari (seafood)—see *Squid*
Camomile (chamomile—herb)—see *Chamomile*
Canadian Bacon (meat)—when diet is completed
Candy (confectionery)—when diet is completed
Cane Sugar (sweetener)—when diet is completed
Cane Syrup (sweetener)—when diet is completed
Cantaloupe (fruit)—Stage III

Cape Gooseberry (fruit)—Stages II & III

Caper (condiment-pickled buds)—Stages II & III, after
introducing vinegar

Carambola (fruit)—Stages II & III

Caraway Seed (seed)—Stages II & III

Cardamom (spice)—Stages II & III

Cardoon (vegetable)—Stages I, II, & III

Caribou (animal)—Stages I, II, & III

Carob (condiment)—when diet is completed

Carp (seafood)—Stages I, II, & III

Carrot (vegetable)—Stages I, II, & III

Carrot Juice (vegetable juice)—Stages II & III

Casaba Melon (fruit)—Stage III

Caserta Squash (vegetable)—Stages I, II, & III

Cashew (nut)—Stages I, II, & III

Cassava (starch)—Stages II & III

Cassis (European black currant syrup)—when diet is completed

Castor Bean (oil)—Stages I, II, & III

Catfish (seafood—all species)—-Stages I, II, & III

Catnip (herb-mint)—fresh in Stage I; dried in Stages II & III

Catsup—see *Ketchup*

Cauliflower (vegetable)—Stages I, II, & III

Caviar (fish eggs)—Stages I, II, & III

Cayenne Pepper (seasoning)—Stages II & III

Celeriac (vegetable)—Stages I, II, & III

Celery (vegetable)—Stages I, II, & III

Celery Knob—see *Celeriac*

Celery Root—see *Celeriac*

Cellophane Noodles (bean threads—mung bean)—Stages II & III

Celery Seed (seed) Stages II & III

Celtuce (vegetable)—Stages I, II, & III

Cereals (grains)—no prepared cereals with sweeteners (barley
malt, corn syrup, rice syrup, sugar, dextrose) until diet is
completed

Challah (hallah, challa—bread)—when diet is completed
Chamomile (herb)—Fresh in Stage I; dried in Stages II & III
Champagne (alcoholic beverage)—when diet is completed
Chapatis—Stages I, II, & III
Chard (vegetable)—Stages I, II, & III
Chayote (fruit)—Stages II & III
Cheese (dairy)—Stage III
Cherry (fruit)—Stages II & III
Chervil (herb)—fresh in Stage I; dried in Stages II & III
Chestnut (nut)—Stage III
Chèvre (goat cheese)—see *Goat Cheese*
Chicken (fowl)—preferably without antibiotics in Stages I, II, &
    III
Chicken broth—fresh in Stages I, II, & III; canned, without
    sweetener or yeast in Stages II & III
Chickpea (garbanzo bean—legume)—Stages I, II, & III
Chicory (blue dandelion, blueweed, coffeeweed, radicchio—
    greens)—Stages I, II, & III
Chili (spice)—fresh in Stage I; dried in Stages II & III
Chili Oil (oil)—Stages I, II, & III
Chili Sauce (sauce)—with fresh tomato only in Stage II; without
    sweetener in Stages II & III
Chinese Cabbage (vegetable)— Stages I, II, & III
Chinese Gooseberry (fruit)—Stages II & III
Chinese Parsley—see *Coriander*
Chinese Potato (vegetable)—Stages I, II, & III
Chinese Preserving Melon (fruit)—Stage III
Chinese Water Chestnut (vegetable)—fresh in Stage I; canned in
    Stages II & III
Chipped Beef (meat)—when diet is completed
Chitterlings (animal intestines)—Stages I, II, & III
Chives (spice)—fresh in Stage I; dried in Stages II & III
Chocolate (confectionery)—when diet is completed
Chorizo (sausage)—when diet is completed

Chowder (soup)—without sweetener in Stages II & III

Chowder Clam (seafood)—Stages I, II, & III

Chub (seafood)—Stages I, II, & III

Chutney (condiment)—when diet is completed

Cider (fermented juice)—see *Apple Cider*

Cilantro—see *Coriander*

Cinnamon (spice)—Stages II & III

Cioppino (seafood soup)—without sweetener in Stages II & III

Cipollini (vegetable)—Stages I, II, & III

Citric Acid (tribasic acid)—when diet is completed

Citron (candied fruit peel)—when diet is completed

Clam (seafood)—Stages I, II, & III

Clove (spice)—Stages II & III

Clover (herb)—see *Honey*

Clover Sprouts (sprouts)—Stages II & III

Cocoa (chocolate—condiment)—when diet is completed

Coconut (fruit)—fresh in Stages II & III; dried when diet is completed

Cod (seafood)—Stages I, II, & III

Coffee (beverage)—when diet is completed

Cola (beverage)—when diet is completed

Collards (vegetable)—Stages I, II, & III

Cole Slaw (cabbage salad)—without sugar in Stages II & III

Comfrey (herb)—fresh in Stage I; dried in Stages II & III

Conserve (fruit/nut jam)—when diet is completed

Consommé (meat broth)—fresh or canned without sweeteners and yeast in Stages I, II, & III

Converted Rice (parboiled rice)—Stage II & III

Cookie (sweet cakes)—when diet is completed

Coriander (spice)—Stages II & III

Corn (vegetable)—Stages I, II, & III

Corn Chip (vegetable)—Stages I, II, & III; whole grain and without yeast and sweeteners

Corn Flour (grain)—undegerminated in Stage I; degerminated in Stages II & III

Cornish Game Hen (meat)—preferably without antibiotics in all Stages

Cornmeal (grain)—fine or coarse; undegermintated in Stage I; degerminated in Stages II & III

Corn Salad (salad greens)—Stages I, II, & III

Corn Starch (starch)—Stages I, II, & III

Corned Beef (brisket of beef—meat)—when diet is completed

Cottage Cheese (dairy)—Stages II & III

Couscous (grain)—Stages II & III

Cowpea (black-eyed peas—legume)—see *Beans*

Crab (seafood)—Stages I, II, & III

Crab Apple (fruit)—Stages II & III

Cracked Wheat (grain)—Stages I, II, & III

Cranberry (fruit)—Stages II & III

Cranberry Bean (legume)—Stages I, II, & III

Crappie (seafood)—Stages I, II, & III

Crayfish (seafood)—Stages I, II, & III

Cream (dairy)—Stages II & III

Cream Cheese (dairy)—Stage III

Cream Sauce (sauce)—Stage II & III

Cream of tartar (baking agent)—Stages I, II, & III

Crenshaw Melon (fruit)—Stage III

Crispbread (unyeasted cracker)—without sweeteners in Stages I, II, & III

Croissant (baked product)—when diet is completed

Crookneck Squash (vegetable)—Stages I, II, & III

Crouton (baked product)—when diet is completed

Cucumber (vegetable)—Stages I, II, & III; avoid skins in I & II

Cumin (spice)—Stages II & III

Curly Cress (greens)—Stages I, II, & III

Currant (fruit)—fresh in Stages II & III; dried when diet is completed

Curry (spice)—Stages II & III

Cushaw Squash (vegetable)—Stages I, II, & III

Cusk (seafood)—Stages I, II, & III

Custard Apple (fruit)—Stages II & III
Cuttlefish (seafood)—Stages I, II, & III

D
Dab (seafood)—Stages I, II, & III
Daikon (vegetable)—Stages I, II, & III
Dandelion (herb)—fresh in Stage I; dried in Stages II & III
Date (dried fruit)—when diet is completed
Date Sugar (sweetener)—when diet is completed
Deer (meat)—Stages I, II, & III
Dextrose (sweetener)—when diet is completed
Dijon Mustard (condiment)—after introducing vinegar, without
    sweetener in Stages II & III
Dill (herb/seed)—fresh in Stage I; dried in Stages II & III
Distilled White Vinegar (vinegar)—Stage II & III
Dolphin fish—see *Mahi Mahi*
Double-Acting Baking Powder—see *Baking Powder*
Dove (fowl)—Stages I, II, & III
Duck (fowl)—Stages I, II, & III
Dulse (seaweed)—fresh in Stage I; dried in Stages II & III

E
Egg (poultry)—preferably without antibiotics in Stages I, II, & III
Eggnog (beverage)—when diet is completed
Eggplant (fruit)—Stages I, II, & III
Eel (seafood)—Stages I, II, & III
Elderberry (fruit)—Stages II & III
Elk (meat)—Stages I, II, & III
Endive (vegetable)—Stages I, II, & III
English Pea (vegetable)—Stages I, II, & III
English Walnut (nut)—Stage III
Enoki mushrooms—see *Mushrooms*
Escarole (vegetable-salad greens)—Stages I, II, & III
Evaporated Milk (dairy canned)—Without sweetener in Stages II
    & III

F

Farina (grain)—Stages II & III

Fava Bean (legume)—Stages I, II, & III

Fennel (vegetable)—Stages I, II, & III

Fennel Seed (seed)—fresh in Stage I; dried in Stages II & III

Fig (fruit)—fresh in Stages II & III; dried when diet is completed

Filbert (nut)—Stages I, II, & III

Filé (sassafras leaves—thickening agent)—fresh in Stage I; dried in Stages II & III

Fish (all types)—Stages I, II, & III

Five-Spice Powder (spice)—Stages II & III

Flageolet (French kidney bean—vegetable)—Stages I, II, & III

Flaxseed (seed & oil)—Stages I, II, & III

Flounder (seafood)—Stages I, II, & III

Flour—see each type listed

Flowers, Edible (condiments)—fresh in Stage I; dried in Stages II & III

Food Additives (additives)—Stages I, II, & III, to be used in moderation

Food Coloring (dyes)—Stages I, II, & III, to be used in moderation

Frankfurter (hot dog, wiener, and frank—meat)—when diet is completed

French Bread (baked product)—without sweetener in Stage III

French Dressing (salad dressing)—without sweetener in Stages II & III

French Endive (vegetable)—Stages I, II, & III

French Fries (potatoes)—with moderation in Stages I, II, & III

French Toast (unyeasted bread, eggs, milk)—without sweeteners in Stages II & III

Fried Rice (grain)—without sweetners in Stages I, II, & III

Fritter (baked grain product)—preferably grains, without sweeteners in Stages I, II, & III

Frog's Legs (seafood)—Stages I, II, & III

Frosting (icing—confectionery)—when diet is completed

Frozen Yogurt (dairy)—with sweetener when diet is completed;
    artifical sweetener in Stages II & III
Fructose (sweetener)—when diet is completed
Fruit Butter (apple or berry spread)—when diet is completed
Fruit—see individual listings
Fruit Juice—for all types, when diet is completed
Fruit Leather (dried fruit)—for all types, when diet is completed
Fudge (confectionery)—when diet is completed
Fuzzy Melon (hairy melon or fuzzy squash—fruit)—Stage III

G
Game Birds (meat)—Stages I, II, & III
Garbanzo (chickpea—legume)—Stages I, II, & III
Garden Pea—see *English Pea*
Garlic (vegetable/spice)—fresh in Stage I; dried in Stages II & III
Garlic Chives (herb)—fresh in Stage I; dried in Stages II & III
Gelatin (thickening agent)—without sweetener in Stages I, II, &
    III
Gherkin (vegetable- pickle)—after vinegar is added back;
    without sweetener in Stages II & III
Gin (alcoholic beverage)—when diet is completed
Ginger (ginger root—condiment/spice)—fresh in Stage I; dried
    in Stages II & III
Ginger Ale (beverage)—artifically sweetened only in Stages I, II,
    & III
Gingerbread (confectionery)—when diet is completed
Ginseng (condiment/herb)—Stages II & III
Globe Artichoke (vegetable)—Stages I, II, & III
Glucose (dextrose, corn sugar, and grape sugar—sweetener)—
    when diet is completed
Gluten Flour (wheat)—Stages II & III
Glycerine (glycerin—additive)—when diet is completed
Gnocchi (pasta)—without cheese in Stages II & III
Goat (meat)—Stages I, II, & III

Goat Cheese (chèvre cheese—cheese)—Stage III

Goats Milk (beverage)—Stages I, II, & III

Golden Nugget Squash (vegetable)—Stages I, II, & III

Goldenrod (herb)—fresh in Stage I; dried in Stages II & III

Golden Seal (herb)—fresh in Stage I; dried in Stages II & III

Golden Syrup (sweetener)—when diet is completed

Goose (fowl)—Stages I, II, & III

Gooseberry (fruit)—Stages II & III

Goosefish—see *Angler*

Graham Flour (wheat)—Stages I, II, & III

Graham Cracker (wheat)—when diet is completed

Granola (grain cereal)—without sweetener and dried fruit, in Stages I, II, & III

Granulated Sugar (sweetener)—see *Sugar*

Grape (fruit)—Stages III

Grape Juice (drink)—when diet is completed

Grapefruit (fruit)—Stages II & III

Grape Sugar (sweetener)—see *Dextrose*

Gravy (meat juices)—using appropriate flour and no wine in Stages I, II, & III

Great Northern Bean (legume)—see *Beans*

Green Beans (vegetable)—Stages I, II, & III

Green Onion (vegetable)—fresh in all stages; dried in Stages II & III

Green Pepper (vegetable)—see *Sweet Pepper*

Green Tea (beverage)—see *Tea-Green*

Grenadine (syrup from pomegranate)—when diet is completed

Grissini (bread sticks)—without sweetener in Stage III

Grits (hominy grits—can be from corn, oats or rice cereal)— Stages II & III

Groats (grain)—Stages II & III

Ground Cherry (Cape gooseberry—fruit)—Stages II & III

Grouper (seafood)—Stages I, II, & III

Grouse (partridge—fowl)—Stages I, II, & III

Grunion (seafood)—Stages I, II, & III

Guacamole (avocado dip)—Stages II & III

Guava (fruit)—Stages II & III

Guinea Fowl (fowl)—Stages I, II, & III

Gunpowder Tea (green tea beverage)—see *Tea, Green*

H

Haddock (seafood)—Stages I, II, & III

Half & Half (dairy)—Stages II & III

Halibut (seafood)—Stages I, II, & III

Ham (meat)—when diet is completed

Hardtack (ship biscuit, sea bread—bread)—Stages I, II, & III

Hash Browns (potatoes)—Stages I, II, & III

Harvest Seafood (seafood)—Stages I, II, & III

Hazelnut (nut)—Stages I, II, & III

Heartnut (nut)—Stage III

Heart of Palm (vegetable)—Stages I, II, & III

Heavy Cream (dairy)—Stages II & III

Herbs (seasoning or medicinal)—fresh in Stage I; dried in Stages II & III, unless taken as part of medical program prescribed by a practitioner

Herring (seafood)—Stages I, II, & III

Hican (nut)—Stage III

Hickory Nut (nut)—Stages I, II, & III

Hog (pork—meat)—fresh in Stages I, II, & III; cured when diet is completed

Hominy (corn)—Stages II & III

Honeydew (fruit)—Stage III

Horehound (medicinal herb)—fresh in Stage I; dried in Stages II & III

Horseradish (condiment)—fresh in Stage I; dried or pickled in Stages II & III

Hot Dog—see *Frankfurter*

Hubbard Squash (vegetable) Stages I, II, & III

Huckleberry (fruit)—Stages I, II, & III

Hummus (garbanzo bean dip)—Stages I, II, & III

Hyssop (herb)—fresh in Stage I; dried in Stages II & III

I

Ice Cream (frozen dairy confectionery)—when diet is completed

Irish Moss (carrageen—seaweed)—fresh in Stage I; dried in
   Stages II & III

Irish Soda Bread (baked grain product)—without sweetener in
   Stages I, II, & III

Italian Sausage (meat)—when diet is completed

Ipe Roxo (tea)—see *Pau d'Arco*

J

Jackfruit (fruit)—Stages II & III

Jam (fruit)—when diet is completed

Jelly (fruit)—when diet is completed

Jerusalem Artichoke (vegetable)—Stages II & III

Jicama (vegetable)—Stages I, II, & III

Juice (drink—all types)—fruit and tomato when diet is
   completed; all other vegetables in Stages II & III

K

Kaki (Japanese persimmon—fruit)—Stages II & III

Kale (vegetable)— Stages I, II, & III

Kamut (grain)—Stages I, II, & III

Kefir (dairy)—without sweetener in Stage III

Kelp (seaweed)—fresh in Stage I; dried in Stages II & III

Ketchup (tomato sauce condiment)—without sweetener and in
   small amounts in Stages II & III

Kidney Bean (legume)—see *Beans*

Kielbasa (meat)—see *Polish Sausage*

Kimchi (spiced cabbage)—without sweeteners in Stages II & III

Kippered Herring (kippers—seafood)—in oil in Stage II; in
   tomato sauce in Stage III

Kiwifruit (Chinese gooseberry—fruit)—Stages II & III

Kohlrabi (vegetable)—Stages I, II, & III

Knackwurst (knockwurst—meat)—when diet is completed

Kumquat (fruit)—Stages II & III

Kuzu (kudzu—starch)—Stages II & III

L

Lady Apple (fruit)—Stages II & III

Lamb (meat)—Stages I, II, & III

Lamb (cheese)—Stage III

Lamb's Quarters (pigweed—salad greens)—Stages I, II, & III

Lamprey (seafood)—Stages I, II, & III

La Pacho (tea)—see *Pau d' Arco*

Lard (pork fat)—Stages II & III

Laurel—see *Bay Leaf*

Lavender (herb)—Fresh in Stage I; dried in Stages II & III

Lecithin (granule or oil)—Stages I, II, & III

Leek (vegetable)—Stages I, II, & III

Legume (beans, peas)—fresh or dried in all Stages; canned, without sweetener in Stages II & III

Lemon (fruit)—half per day in Stage I; unlimited in Stages II & III

Lemon Juice (drink)—without sweetener in Stages I, II, & III

Lemon Balm (herb)—fresh in Stage I; dried in Stages II & III

Lemon Grass (herb)—fresh in Stage I; dried in Stages II & III

Lemon Verbena (herb)—fresh in Stage I; dried in Stages II & III

Lentil (legume)—Stages I, II, & III

Lettuce (greens)—Stages I, II, & III

Licorice (herb)—fresh in Stage I; dried in Stages II & III

Lima Bean (legume)—Stages I, II, & III

Lime (fruit)—Stages I, II, & III

Limpet (seafood)—Stages I, II, & III

Lingcod (Greenling—seafood)—Stages I, II, & III

Lingonberry (fruit)—fresh, without sweetener in Stages II & III

Linguica (sausage)—without sweetener in Stages II & III

Liquor (alcholic beverage)—when diet is completed

Litchi (lychee—fruit)—Stages II & III

Liver (meat)—Stages I, II, & III; eat only organic or young animal
  organs
Liverwurst (meat)—see *Sandwich Meat*
Lobster (seafood)—Stages I, II, & III
Loganberry (fruit)—Stages II & III
Longberry (fruit)—Stages II & III
Loquat (fruit)—Stages II & III
Lovage (herb)—fresh in Stage I; dried in Stages II & III
Lychee (fruit)—see *Litchi*

M

Macadamia (Queensland—nut)—Stages I, II, & III
Mace (spice)—Stages II & III
Mackerel (seafood)—Stages I, II, & III
Mahi mahi (dolphin fish—seafood)—Stages I, II, & III
Malanga (West Indian kale—herb)—fresh in Stage I; dried in
  Stages II & III
Malt (sweetener)—when diet is completed
Malto Dextrin (sweetener)—when diet is completed
Malt Vinegar (vinegar)—Stages II & III
Maltose (malt sugar—sweetener)—when diet is completed
Mandarin Orange (fruit)—Stages II & III
Mango (fruit)—Stages II & III
Maple Sugar or Syrup (sweetener)—when diet is completed
Margarine—Stages I, II, & III
Marjoram (herb/spice)—fresh in Stage I, dried in Stages II & III
Marmalade (jam)—when diet is completed
Marlin (seafood)—Stages I, II, & III
Marshmallow (confectionery)—when diet is completed
Marzipan (confectionery)—when diet is completed
Masa Harina (grain—corn)—Stages II & III
Maté (yerba de maté—herb)—fresh in Stage I; dried in Stages II
  & III
Matzo (matzoh—unleavened bread)—plain in Stage I; with
  dried herbs on Stages II & III

Mayonnaise (dressing)—after vinegar is added in Stages II & III
Melon (fruit)—all types in Stage III
Milk, Cow (dairy)—Stages II & III
Milk, Goat (dairy)—Stages II & III
Millet (grain)—Stages I, II, & III
Milo (grain)—Stages I, II, & III
Mineral Water (beverage)—plain only in Stages I, II, & III
Mint (herb)—fresh in Stage I; dried in Stages II & III
Miso (soybean paste)—Stages II & III
Mocha (beverage)—when diet is completed
Mochi (sweet rice product)—plain or mugwort flavors only in
    Stage III
Molasses (sweetener)—when diet is completed
Monkfish (angler—seafood)—Stages I, II, & III
Monosodium Glutamate (MSG)—when diet is completed
Moose (meat)—Stages I, II, & III
Morel (fungus—mushroom)—Stage III
Mortadella (smoked sausage)—when diet is completed
Muesli (cereal)—when diet is completed
Muffin (baked product)—using appropriate form of grain,
    without sweetener in Stages I, II, & III; with fruit in Stages II
    & III
Mugicha (toasted whole barley)—Stages I, II, & III
Mulberry (fruit)—Stages II & III
Mullet (seafood)—Stages I, II, & III
Mung Bean (legume)—Stages I, II, & III
Muscadine (fruit—grape)—Stage III
Muscat Grape (fruit)—Stage III
Mush (cooked cereal)—using the appropriate form of grain,
    without sweetener in Stages I, II, & III; with milk in Stages II
    & III
Mushroom (fungus—mushroom)—Stage III
Muskmelon (fruit)—Stage III
Mussel (seafood)—Stages I, II, & III
Mustard (condiment)—without sweetener or wine; after adding

vinegar, in Stages II & III
Mustard Greens (vegetable)—Stages I, II, & III
Mustard Seed (spice)—Stages II & III
Mutton (meat)—Stages I, II, & III

N
Napa Cabbage (Chinese Cabbage—vegetable) Stages I, II, & III
Nasturtium (edible flower and leaves)—Stages I, II, & III
Navy Bean (legume)—see *Beans*
Nectarine (fruit)—Stages II & III
New Zealand Spinach (vegetable)—Stages I, II, & III
Noodle (pasta)—whole grain in Stage I; any type in Stages II & III
Nori (seaweed)—fresh in Stage I; dried in Stages II & III
Nutmeg (spice)—Stages II & III
Nutritional Yeast (supplement)—see *Yeast*
Nuts—see individual listings

O
Oat (groats—grain)—Stages I, II, & III
Oats, Old-Fashioned (grain)—Stages I, II, & III
Oats, Quick-Cooking (grain)—Stages II & III
Oats, Scotch, or Steel-Cut or Irish (grain)—Stages I, II, & III
Oatmeal (grain)—Stages I, II, & III
Oatmeal, Instant—without sweetener in Stages II & III
Oat Bran (grain)—Stages I, II, & III
Oat Flour (grain)—Stages I, II, & III
Ocean Catfish (fish)—Stages I, II, & III
Ocean Perch (fish)—Stages I, II, & III
Octopus (seafood)—Stages I, II, & III
Oils —almond, avocado, canola, corn, hazelnut, olive, pumpkin seed, safflower, sesame, soy, sunflower, palm kernel, walnut and wheat germ—in all Stages; peanut oil in Stage III.
Okra (vegetable)—Stages I, II, & III
Olallieberry (fruit)—Stages II & III

Olive (condiment)—Stages II & III

Olive Oil—see *Oil*

Onion (vegetable)—fresh in Stage I; dried or powdered in II & III

Orange (fruit)—Stages II & III

Orange Juice (drink)—when diet is completed

Orange Roughy (seafood)—Stages I, II, & III

Oregano (herb)— Fresh in Stage I; dried in Stages II & III

Oyster (seafood)—Stages I, II, & III

Oyster Plant (salsify—root vegetable)—Stages I, II, & III

P

Pak Choi (vegetable)—see *Bok Choy*

Palm Cabbage (edible bud of the palm tree—fruit)—Stages II & III

Pancake (baked product)—using appropriate flour, without sweeteners in Stages I, II, & III

Pancetta (Italian bacon)—when diet is completed

Papaya (fruit)—Stages II & III; dried when diet is completed

Paprika (spice)—Stages II & III

Paradise Nut (sapucaya nut—nut)—Stages II & III

Parsley (herb/salad greens)—fresh in Stage I; dried in Stages II & III

Parsnip (vegetable)—Stages I, II, & III

Partridge (fowl)—see *Grouse*

Passion Fruit (fruit)—Stages II & III

Pastry Flour (grain)—whole wheat Stage I; white Stage II & III

Pasta (noodles)—using appropriate flour in Stages I, II, & III

Pastrami (meat)—see *Sandwich Meat*

Pattypan Squash (vegetable)—Stages I, II, & III

Paté (ground-meat preparation)—without wine or sweeteners in Stages II & III

Pau d'Arco (Bow Stick, Ipe Roxo, La Pacho, Quaw Bark, Taheebo and Tecoma—antifungal bark tea)—Stages I, II, & III

Pawpaw (fruit)—Stages II & III

Pea (vegetable—legume)—Stages I, II, & III

Peafowl (fowl)—Stages I, II, & III

Peach (fruit)—Stages II & III; dried when diet is completed

Peach Juice (drink)—when diet is completed

Peanut (nut)—Stage III

Peanut Butter (nut butter spread)—without sweetener in Stage III

Pear (fruit)—Stages II & III; dried when diet is completed

Pear juice (drink)—when diet is completed

Pearl Barley—see *Barley*

Pecan (nut)—Stages I, II, & III

Pectin (fruit starch)—Stages II & III

Pennyroyal (herb)—fresh in Stage I; dried in Stages II & III

Pepper, sweet (vegetable)—Stages I, II, & III

Pepper (capsicum, hot—spice)—fresh in Stage I; dried in Stages II & III

Peppercorn (spice) —see *Black Pepper*

Peppermint (herb)—fresh in Stage I; dried in Stages II & III

Pepperoni (meat)—when diet is completed

Perch (all types—seafood)—Stages I, II, & III

Persian Melon (fruit)—Stage III

Persimmon (fruit)—Stages II & III

Pheasant (fowl)—Stages I, II, & III

Pickles (condiment)—Stages II & III

Pickerel (seafood)—Stages I, II, & III

Picnic Ham (meat)—when diet is completed

Pigeon (squab—fowl)—Stages I, II, & III

Pike (seafood)—Stages I, II, & III

Pimenta (allspice)—dried in Stages II & III

Pimiento (vegetable)—fresh in Stage I; pickled in Stages II & III

Pineapple (fruit)—Stages II & III; dried when diet is completed

Pinenut (nut)—Stages I, II, & III

Pinto Bean (legume)—see *Beans*

Pistachio (nut)—Stage III

Pita Bread (yeasted baked product)—without sweetener in Stage III

Pizza (baked product)—without sweeteners in Stage III

Plaice (seafood)—Stages I, II, & III

Plantain (fruit)—fresh in Stages II & III; dried when diet is completed

Plum (fruit)—Stages II & III

Polenta (cornmeal)—Stages II & III

Poi (dasheen, taro root—starch)—Stages II & III

Polish Sausage (meat)—when diet is completed

Pollack (pollock—seafood)—Stages I, II, & III

Pomegranate (fruit)—Stages II & III

Pompano (seafood)—Stages I, II, & III

Popcorn (grain)—Stages I, II, & III

Poppyseed (seed)—Stages I, II, & III

Pork (meat)— fresh only and preferrably without antibiotics in Stages I, II, & III; cured when diet is completed

Potato (vegetable)—Stages I, II, & III; avoid skins in Stages I & II

Potato Chips (fried vegetable)—without sweetener in Stages I, II, & III

Pot Cheese (dairy)—Stage II & III

Poultry (meat)—preferably without antibiotics in Stages I, II, & III; avoid eating skin

Powdered Milk (dairy)—Stages II & III

Prawn (seafood)—Stages I, II, & III

Pretzel (baked cracker)—when diet is completed

Prickly Pear (fruit)—Stages II & III

Prosciutto (Italian ham)—when diet is completed

Prune (dried plums—fruit)—when diet is completed

Pumpkin (fruit)—Stages II & III

Pumpkin Seeds (pepitas—seeds)—Stages I, II, & III

Pumpkinseed (sunfish—sea food) Stages I, II, & III

Q
Quail (fowl)—Stages I, II, & III

Quaw Bark (tea)—see *Pau d'Arco*

Queensland Nut (macadamia—nut)—Stages I, II, & III

Quince (fruit)—Stages II & III
Quinoa (grain)—Stages I, II, & III

R

Rabbit (meat)—Stages I, II, & III
Radish (vegetable)—Stages I, II, & III
Raisin (fruit)—when diet is completed
Ramen (noodles)—without sweetener in Stages II & III
Raspberry (fruit)—Stage III
Red Pepper (vegetable)—Stages I, II, & III
Red Snapper (seafood)—Stages I, II, & III
Rhubarb (vegetable)—without sweetener in Stages I, II, & III
Rice (grain)—whole grain, brown rice in Stage I; processed or
    white rice in Stages II & III
Rice Cakes—without sweetener in Stages I, II, & III; without
    sweetener with cheese in Stage III
Rice Vinegar (vinegar)—Stages II & III
Ricotta Cheese (dairy)—Stage III
Risotto (Italian rice)—Stages II & III
Rock Fish (seafood)—Stages I, II, & III
Roe (fish eggs)—Stages I, II, & III
Romaine (greens)—Stages I, II, & III
Rosehips (herb)—Stages II & III
Rosemary (herb)— fresh in Stage I; dried in Stages II & III
Rutabaga (Swede—vegetable)—Stages I, II, & III
Rye (grain)—Stages I, II, & III

S

Saccharin (artificial sweetener)—Stages I, II, & III; to be used in
    moderation
Saffron (spice)—Stages II & III
Sage (herb)—fresh in Stage I; dried in Stages II & III
Sailfish (seafood)—Stages I, II, & III
Salami (meat)—when diet is completed
Salmon (seafood)—Stages I, II, & III

Salsify (vegetable)—see *Oyster Plant*

Salt (seasoning)—Stages I, II, & III

Sandwich Meats (prepared meats)—when diet is completed

Sardine (seafood)—in oil, Stages I, II, & III; in tomato sauce in Stage III

Sarsaparilla (root beer—herb)—fresh in Stage I; dried in Stages II & III

Sashimi (raw fish)—when diet is completed

Sassafras (filé—thickening agent)—fresh in Stage I; dried in Stages II & III

Sauces (preparded condiments)—no vinegar, without sweetener, or with yeast in Stages I, II, & III

Sauerkraut (fermented cabbage)—Stages II & III

Sauger (perch—seafood)—Stages I, II, & III

Sausage (meat)—when diet is complete

Savory (herb)—fresh in Stage I; dried in Stages II & III

Scallion (onion—vegetable)—Stages I, II, & III

Scallop (seafood)— Stages I, II, & III

Scone (baked product)—using appropriate flour, without sweetener in Stages I, II, & III

Scotch Oats (grain)—Stages I, II, & III

Sea Bass (seafood)—Stages I, II, & III

Sea Herring (seafood)—fresh in Stages I, II, & III; pickled in Stages II & III

Sea Trout (seafood)—Stages I, II, & III

Seaweed (algae)—Stages I, II, & III

Seckel Pear (fruit)—Stages II & III

Sesame (seed)—Stages I, II, & III

Shad (seafood)—Stages I, II, & III

Shallot (vegetable)—Stages I, II, & III

Shark (seafood)—Stages I, II, & III

Sheep (lamb—meat)—Stages I, II, & III

Shellfish (seafood)—Stages I, II, & III

Shrimp (seafood)—Stages I, II, & III

Smelt (seafood)—Stages I, II, & III

Smoked meat or fish—without sweeteners in Stages II & III

Snail (mollusk)—Stages I, II, & III

Snapper (seafood)—Stages I, II, & III

Snow Pea (Chinese snow peas, sugar peas—vegetable)—Stages II & III

Sole (seafood)—Stages I, II, & III

Sorbitol (artificial sweetener)—Stages I, II, & III, to be used in moderation

Sorghum (syrup—sweetener)—when diet is completed

Sorrel (herb)—Fresh in Stage I; dried in Stages II & III

Soup (prepared, fresh, or canned)—fresh or canned without tomato in Stages I & II; canned with tomato in Stage III; all Stages without sweeteners

Sour Cream (dairy)—Stage III

Sourdough (starter for bread)—Stage III, without sweetener

Soybean (legume)—see *Beans*

Soy Flour (legume—flour)—Stages I, II, & III

Soy Milk (legume—beverage)—without sweetener in Stages I, II, & III

Soy Sauce (legume—sauce)—without sweetener or MSG in Stages II & III

Spaghetti (grain—pasta)—using appropriate grain in Stages I, II, & III

Spaghetti Squash (vegetable)—Stages I, II, & III

Spanish Melon (fruit)—Stage III

Spearmint (herb)—fresh in Stage I; dried in Stages II & III

Spelt (grain)—Stages I, II, & III

Spices (seasoning)—fresh in Stage I; dried in Stage II & III

Spinach (vegetable)—Stages I, II, & III

Spotted Sea Trout (seafood)—Stages I, II, & III

Squab (pigeon)—Stages I, II, & III

Squash (vegetable—all varieties)—Stages I, II, & III

Squid (seafood)—Stages I, II, & III

Star Anise (spice)—fresh in Stage I; dried in Stage II & III

Stevia (sweetner—herb)—when diet is completed

Stock (meat, fish or vegetable)—fresh or canned without sweetener in Stages I, II, & III; dried without sweetener in Stage II

Strawberry (fruit)—Stages II & III

String Bean (vegetable)—Stages I, II, & III

Sturgeon (seafood)—Stages I, II, & III

Sucker (seafood)—Stages I, II, & III

Sucrose (sweetener)—when diet is completed

Sugar Beet (sweetener)—when diet is completed

Sugar Cane (sweetener)—when diet is completed

Summer Savory (herb)--fresh in Stage I; dried in Stages II & III

Sunfish (seafood)—Stages I, II, & III

Sunflower Seeds (seeds)—Stages I, II, & III

Sushi Rice (grain)—Stages II & III

Sweet Brown Rice (grain)—Stages II & III

Sweet Cicely (herb)—fresh in Stage I; dried in Stages II & III

Sweet Corn (vegetable)—Stages I, II, & III

Sweet Pepper (bell pepper—vegetable)—Stages I, II, & III

Sweet Potato (vegetable)—Stages I, II, & III

Swordfish (seafood)—Stages I, II, & III

T

Tabbouleh (bulghur wheat salad)—with fresh ingredients only on Stage I; dried in Stages II & III

Taheebo (tea)—see *Pau d'Arco*

Tahini (sesame seed butter)—Stages I, II, & III

Tamarind (fruit)—Stages II & III

Tangelo (fruit)—Stages II & III

Tangerine (fruit)—Stages II & III

Tansy (herb)—fresh in Stage I; dried in Stages II & III

Tapioca (starch)—without sweetener in Stages II & III

Taro (poi, dasheen—starch)—Stages II & III

Tarragon (herb)—fresh in Stage I; dried in Stages II & III

Tartar Sauce (condiment)—without sweetener in Stages II & III

Tea, Black (beverage)—when diet is completed

Tea, Green (beverage)—Hoji-cha, Stage II; all others when diet is completed

Tea, Herbal (tisane—beverage)—fresh in Stage I; dried in Stages II & III

Tea Melon (fruit)—Stage III

Tecoma (tea)—see *Pau d'Arco*

Teff (grain)—Stages I, II, & III

Tempeh (fermented soy product)—Stages II & III

Tequila (cactus plant—distilled spirits)—when diet is completed

Texmati Rice (grain)—white in Stages II & III ; brown in Stages I, II, & III

Thyme (herb)—fresh in Stage I; dried in Stages II & III

Tilefish (seafood)—Stages I, II, & III

Tofu (soybean curd)—Stages II & III; don't store in refrigerator for more than 3 days; change storage water daily

Tomatillo (fruit)—Stages II & III

Tomato (fruit)—fresh in Stages I, II, & III; canned, without sweeteners in Stage III

Tomato Juice (vegetable juice)—when diet is completed

Tomato Sauce—fresh in Stages I, II, & III; canned without sweeteners, Stage III

Tonic Water (beverage)—with artificial sweetener in Stages I, II, & III

Tortillas (corn or wheat product)—Stage I, whole grains; Stage II & III, processed grains

Triticale (grain)—Stages II & III

Trout (seafood)—Stages I, II, & III

Truffle (fungus)—Stage III

Tuna (seafood)—fresh in Stage I ; canned, water-packed in Stages II & III

Turbot (seafood)—Stages I, II, & III

Turkey (fowl)—preferably without antibiotics in Stages I, II, & III

Turmeric (spice)—Stages II & III

Turnip (vegetable)—Stages I, II, & III
TVP (textured vegetable protein)—Stages II & III

U
Upland Cress (salad greens)—Stages I, II, & III

V
Vanilla (spice)—dried bean in Stage II & III, extract when diet is completed
Vanillin (artifical spice)—when diet is completed
Veal (meat)—Stages I, II, & III
Vegetables—see individual listings
Venison (meat)—Stages I, II, & III (55)
Vermicelli (pasta)—Stage II & III
Vinegar (condiment)—Stages II & III (see specific types)

W
Waffle (baked product)—using appropriate grains, without sweeteners in Stages I, II, & III
Walleye (seafood)—Stages I, II, & III
Walnuts (Black or English—nut)—Stage III
Wasabi (wasabe—horseradish)—Stages II & III
Water Chestnut (vegetable)—fresh in Stage I; canned in water in Stages II & III
Watercress (greens)—Stages I, II, & III
Watermelon (fruit)—Stage III
Weakfish (seafood)—Stages I, II, & III
Wehani Rice (grain)—Stages I, II, & III
Wheat (grain)—-whole grains in Stage I; processed grains in Stages II & III
Wheat Germ (grain)—Stages I, II, & III
Whitebait (seafood)—Stages I, II, & III
White Beans (legumes)—see *Beans*
Whitefish (seafood)—Stages I, II, & III
White Pepper (spice)—Stages I, II, & III
White Perch (seafood)—Stages I, II, & III

White Walnut—see *Butternut*

Whiting (seafood)—Stages I, II, & III

Wild Rice (grain)—Stages I, II, & III

Wine—see *Alcohol*

Wintergreen (flavoring, not oil)—without alcohol and sweetener in Stages I, II, & III

Winter Melon (fruit)—Stage III

Winter Savory (herb)—fresh in Stage I; dried in Stages II & III

Witloof Chicory—see *French Endive*

Woodruff (herb)—fresh in Stage I; dried in Stages II & III

Worcestershire Sauce (condiment)—when diet is completed

X

Xanthan Gum (from fermented corn sugar—thickener)—Stage II & III

Y

Yam (vegetable)—Stages I, II, & III

Yarrow (herb)—fresh in Stage I; dried in Stages II & III

Yautia (starch)—Stages II & III

Yeast (Baker's, Brewer's, or nutritional)—without sweetener in Stage III

Yellow Bass (seafood)—Stages I, II, & III

Yellow Jack (seafood)—Stages I, II, & III

Yellow Perch (seafood)—Stages I, II, & III

Yerba Maté—see *Maté*

Yogurt (dairy)—plain with live cultures, without sweeteners or fruit in Stages I, II, & III

Youngberry (fruit)—Stages II & III

Yuca (cassava—starch)—Stages II & III

Z

Zucchini (vegetable)—Stages I, II, & III

Zwieback (twiced-baked product)—whole grain, without sweetener in Stages I, II, & III

Appendices

Sources for Nutritional Supplements
and Antifungal Preparations

THE FOLLOWING SUPPLIERS carry many of the antifungal preparations previously mentioned in the book, as well as other
healthful products. All of these companies deal with health food
stores or practitioners rather than directly with consumers. If there
is a product you would like to try, ask your doctor/health practitioner, local pharmacy, or health food store to help you order it. Or
call the suppliers listed and find out if there is a local person or store
in your area already using the product and go to them directly.

Alacer Corporation, 14 Morgan, Irvine, CA 92718; 800-854-0249
    Makes a wonderful unsweetened version of a product called
Emergen-C, which has electrolytes, potassium, and Vitamin C in
individual easy-to-carry packages.

Allergy Alternative, 440 Godfrey Drive, Windsor, CA 95492-8036; 800-
838-1514/707-838-1514
    A mail-order company specializing in a diverse line of enviro-
mentally safe products at discounted prices. Offers vitamins, acidophilus, and antifungals as well as personal care products.

Allergy Research Group/Nutricology, 400 Preda Street, San Leandro,
CA 94577; 800-545-9960
    A nutritional supplement company for chemically sensitive/aller-
gic people. Good quality products for multiple vitamins/minerals
as well as digestive enzymes.

bio/chem Research, 865 Parallel Drive, Lakeport, CA 95453; 800-225-
4345
    Provides a grapefruit seed extract called Citricidal (see page 56).

Bronson Pharmaceuticals, P. O. Box 628, La Cañada, CA 91012; 800-521-3322
 Has a reasonably priced line of supplements for the whole family including Vitamin C crystals without sodium.

Cardiovascular Research/Ecological Formulas, 1061-B Shary Circle, Concord, CA 94518; 800-888-4585/510-827-2636
 Makes Orithrush products along with other formulas for immune support, yeast problems and allergies (see page 54).

DaVinci Laboratories/Food Science Laboratories, 20 New England Drive, Essex Junction, VT 05453; 800-325-1776
 Carries a reputable line of nutritional products including DMG (N-N dimethylglycine).

Dolisos America, Inc., 3014 Rigel Avenue, Las Vegas, NV 89102; 800-365-4767
 A full-service homeopathic company featuring a fairly complete family first-aid kit.

Ecological Formulas (see *Cardiovascular Research*)

Enzymatic Therapy, P. O. Box 1508, Green Bay, WI 54305; 800-558-7372
 Produces a wide range of good-quality nutritional, naturopathic, herbal, and glandular remedies.

Freeda, 36 E 41st Street, New York, N.Y. 10017; 800-777-3737
 Offers a wide range of products for the whole family that are vegetarian and free of aluminum, coal tar dyes, and yeast.

K'an Herb, 2425 Porter Street, Ste. 18, Soquel, CA 95073; 408-462-9915
 Makes herbal products for acupuncturists and health care professionals, including a collection of bio-radiance products (Biocidin, Biotonic, Bio-Radiance used as antifungals), along with echinacea and Pau d'Arco (see page 57).

Karuna Corporation, 42 Digital Drive, #7, Novato, CA 94949; 800-826-7225

Makes excellent digestive enzymes along with multiple vitamin-minerals and glandulars; carries an assortment of effective nutrient products like CoQ_{10}, acidophilus, and echinacea (see page 62).

Klaire Laboratories/Vital Life, 1537 W Seminole, San Marcos, CA 92069; 800-533-7255

Carries hypo-allergenic acidophilus called Vita Plex and Vita Dophilus which work well in the colon.

Metegenics, Inc., 971 Calle Negocio, San Clemente, CA 92672; 800-692-9400

Offers an excellent group of products with a separated acidophilus and bifidus, better for digestion; exclusively carries Ultra Balance (see page 62).

National CFIDS Buyers Catalog, 1187 Coast Village Road, #1-280, Santa Barbara, CA 93108; 800-366-6056

Mail order company carring CoQ_{10}, garlic, golden seal, echinacea, acidophilus, digestive enzymes, evening primrose oil, as well as many other nutritional products at discount prices.

Natren, 3105 Willow Lane, Westlake Village, CA 91361; 800-992-3323, 800-992-9393 in California

Specializes in acidophilus and bifus products. An improved adhesion strain of acidophilus is called "Bio-Nate."

Nature's Plus, 10 Daniel Street, Farmingdale, NY 11735; 800-937-0500

Offers yeast-free B vitamins as well as multi-vitamins; products commonly found in natural food stores.

Nature's Way Products, Inc., 10 Mountain Springs Parkway, Springville, UT 84663; 800-453-1468

Carries evening primrose oil, liquid chlorophyll, and other nutritional products.

N.E.E.D.S., 527 Charles Avenue, 12-A, Syracuse, NY 13209; 800-634-1380
Mail order discount company specializing in multivitamins and some antifungal products like caprylic acid, citrus seed extract, and acidophilus (see page 57).

NF Formulas, Inc., 805 S.E. Sherman, Portland, OR 97214; 800-547-4891
Carries naturopathic products including vitamin C and echinacea.

Nutricology (see *Allergy Research Group*)

Nutri-Dyn, 222 N Vincent Avenue, Covina, CA 91722; 800-327-8355
Offers a good line of glandular products as well as other nutritional products.

Nutrition Resource, P. O. Box 238, Lakeport, CA 95453; 800-225-4345
Makes hypo-allergenic supplements with a reasonably priced vitamin C powder.

Nutriwest, 27 Mauchly, #205, Irvine, CA 92718; 800-541-1588
Has a wonderful product called Molybdenum, which is good for immune compromised or allergic people.

Probiologic, Inc., 14714 NE 87th Street, Redmond, WA 98052; 800-678-8218
Makers of Capricin and other professional nutritional products.

Scientific Consulting Service, 466 Whitney Street, San Leandro, CA 94577; 800-333-7414
Supplies Germanium and Tannalbit as well as other nutritional products.

Terrace International, 10 Mountain Spring Parkway, Springville, UT 84663; 800-824-2434
Carries Cantrol and Citronex, citrus seed extract (see page 56).

Twin Labs, 2120 Smithtown Avenue, Ronkonkoma, NY 11779; 800-645-5626
Has an excellent yeast-free product line of vitamins and minerals available in health food stores.

Vitamin Express, 1425 Irving Street, San Francisco, CA 94122; 415-564-8160
Has two stores and is also equipped for mail orders. Includes a very nice assortment of antifungal products with discounted prices and very helpful with information.

Wellness Health Pharmaceuticals, 2800 S 18th Street, Birmingham, AL 35209; 800-227-2672
Mail order distributor for many nutritional and pharmaceutical products including Nystatin powder and some other Candida therapy products.

Yerba Prima, P. O. Box 2569, Oakland, CA 94614; 800-421-9972
Provides an intestinal cleansing program with herbs; also carries excellent echinacea tablets.

Mail Order Food Sources

Allergy Resources, P. O. Box 888 Brookridge, Palmer Lake, CO 80133; 719-488-3630

Carries organic, whole grain pastas and flours, including teff and a yeast-free brown rice bread.

Arrowhead Mills, P. O. Box 2059, Hereford, TX 79045; 800-749-0730 (for mail order catalog)/806-364-0730
Will mail any amount from their catalog; carries teff flour along with many other whole foods.

Bob's Red Mill, Milwaukie, OR 97222
For xanthan gum. Write for a catalog.

Coleman Natural Beef, Denver, CO 80251-0131; 800-442-8668 (for mail order catalog)
Reliable, large company that carries all kinds of cuts and will send any amount. Your butcher or meat department may be interested in carrying this company's product.

The 1994 National Directory of Organic Wholesalers, California Action Network, P. O. Box 464, Davis, CA 95617; 916-756-8518
Has a complete listing of organic wholesalers across the U.S. along with a mail order section to the general public.

Organic Veal by Matt Doerksen, 209-634-6889/209-634-9981
Individual orders accepted by phone only; supplies are very limited.

Special Foods, 9207 Shotgun Court, Springfield, VA 22153; 703-644-0991
Has a complete line of breads, pastas, flours and crackers all made from roots instead of grains.

Texas Wild Game Cooperative, P. O. Box 530, Ingram, TX 78025; 800-962-4263
Mail order for antibiotic-free venison, antelope, wild boar, and wild boar sausage.

Vegetarian Lifestyle, Harvest Direct, Inc., P. O. Box 4514, Decatur, IL 62525-4514; 800-835-2867/217-422-3324

Carries whole wheat couscous, brown basmati rice, brown rice pasta and organic wild rice, as well as many other items.

Candida Practioners

American Academy of Environmental Medicine (formerly the Society for Clinical Ecology), P. O. Box 16106, Denver, CO 80216; 303-622-9755

Can send you a nationwide list of M.D.s who practice Candida therapy, as well as environmental medicine.

American Association of Acupuncturists, 4101 Lake Boone Trail, Suite 201, Raleigh, NC 27607

Will provide general licensed referrals in a three-state area. Send written requests with $5.00 and the three states from which you want referrals. Interview carefully to make sure the practioner is familiar with Candida therapy.

American Association of Naturopathic Physicians, 2366 Eastlake Avenue E, #322, Seattle, WA 948102

Will give a general referral for Naturopath doctors throughout the U.S. Send a self-addressed, stamped envelope to the address above for a list in your area.

Great Smokies Lab Client Services; 800-522-4762

Test for Candida, as well as parasites in stool and serum. Will direct you to a practioner in your area that does Candida therapy.

Meridan Labs, 24030-132nd Avenue SE, Kent, WA 98042; 206-631-8922

Provides comprehensive stool analysis for digestion and Candida albicans. Will direct you to a practioner in your area that does Candida therapy.

Bibliography

Airola, Paavo. *How to Get Well.* Phoenix, AZ: Health Plus, 1974

Balch, James F., and Phyllis Balch. *A Prescription for Nutritional Healing.* Garden City Park, New York: Avery Publishing, 1990.

Ballentine, Rudolph. *Diet and Nutrition.* Honesdale, PA: Himalayan Publishers, 1978.

Berger, Stuart M. *Dr. Berger's ImmunePower Diet.* New York: Signet Books, 1986.

Bland, Jeffrey. *Nutraerobics.* San Francisco: Harper & Row, 1985. O.P.
_____ *Trace Elements in Human Health and Disease.* Redmond, WA: Eagle Print, 1979. O.P.

Bricklin, Mark, and staff. *The Natural Healing Annual.* Emmaus, PA: Rodale Press, 1987.

Brody, Jane. *Jane Brody's Nutrition Book.* New York: Bantam Books, 1982.

Brostoff, J., and L. Gammlin. *The Complete Guide to Food Allergy and Intolerance.* London: Bloomsbury, 1989.

Burtis, Grace, Judi Davis and Sandra Martin. *Applied Nutrition and Diet Therapy.* Philadelphia, PA: W. B. Saunders, 1988.

Colbin, Annemarie. *Food and Healing.* New York: Ballantine Books, 1986.

Crook, William. *The Yeast Connection.* New York: Vintage Books, 1986.

_____ *Detecting Your Hidden Food Allergies.* Jackson, TN: Professional Books, 1988.

_____ *Chronic Fatigue Syndrome and the Yeast Connection.* Jackson, TN: Professional Books, 1992.

Diamond, Harvey, and Marilyn Diamond. *Fit for Life.* New York: Warner Books, 1987.

Dumke, Nicolette, M. *Allergy Cooking With Ease.* Lancaster, PN: Starburst Publishers, 1992.

Hertigage, Ford. *Composition and Facts About Foods.* Moelumne Hill, CA: Health Research, 1971.

Garrison, Robert H., Jr., and Eliabeth Somer. *Nutrition Desk Reference.* New Canaan, CT: Keats Publishing, 1985.

Golos, Natalie, and Frances G. Golos. *Coping With Your Allergies.* New York: Simon and Schuster, 1986.

Golos, Natalie, James F. O'Shea, Francis J. Waickman, and Frances G. Golbitz. *Enviornmental Medicine.* New Cannan: Keats Publishing, 1987.

Haas, Elson M. *Staying Healthy with Nutrition.* Berkeley, CA: Celestial Arts, 1992.

Herbst, Sharon T. *Food Lover's Companion.* Hauppauge, NY: Barron's, 1990.

Hunter, Beatrice *The Great Nutrition Robbery.* New York: Charles Scribner's Sons, 1978.

King, Jonathan. *Troubled Water: The Poisoning of America's Drinking Water.* Emmaus, PA: Rodale Press, 1985.

Lark, Susan. *Premenstrual Syndrome Self-Help Book.* Berkeley, CA: Celestial Arts, 1989.

Levin, Alan S., and Merla Zellerbach. *Type 1/Type 2 Allergy Relief Program.* Los Angeles, CA: Jeremy Tarcher, 1983.

Margen, Sheldon, and editors. *The Wellness Encyclopedia of Food and Nutrition.* New York: Rebus, 1992.

Murray, Michael, and Joseph Pizzorno. *An Encyclopedia of Natural Medicine.* Rocklin, CA: Prima Publishing, 1991.

Pelletier, Kenneth R. *Mind As Healer Mind As Slayer.* New York: Delta Books, 1987.

Pemberton Cindy, and Marcia Brown. *The Creative Eater's Handbook —Better Nutrition Through Vegetarian Eating.* Oakland, CA: American Heart Association, 1983.

Pennington, Jean A. T. *Food Values of Portions Commonly Used, 15th Edition.* New York: Perennial Library, 1989.

Randolph, Theron G., and Ralph W. Moss. *An Alternative Approach to Allergies: The New Field of Clinical Ecology Unravels the Environ-*

mental Causes of Mental and Physical Ills, Revised Edition. New York: Perennial Library, 1990.

Rapp, Doris J. *Allergies and Your Family.* New York: Publisher's Press, 1990.

Remington, Dennis W., and Barbara W. Higa. *Back To Health.* Provo, Utah: Vitality House International, 1986.

Rinkel, Herbert J. *The Management of Clinical Allergy.* Cheyenne, WY: Russel I Williams, M. D., 1983.

Robbins, John. *Diet for a New America: How Your Food Choices Affect Your Health, Happiness and Future of Life on Earth.* Walpole, NH: Stillpoint Publishing, 1987.

Rodale Press Editors. *The Complete Book of Vitamins.* Emmaus, PA: Rodale Press, 1984. O. P.

Rose, Jeannie. *Herbs and Things: Jeanne Rose's Herbal.* New York: Grossett and Dunlap, 1972.

Russell-Manning, Betsy. *Home Remedies For Candida, 3rd Edition.* San Francisco, CA: Greensward Press, 1989.

Saifer, Phyllis, and Merla Zellerbach. *Detox.* Los Angeles, CA: Jeremy P. Tarcher, 1984.

Truss, C. Orian. *The Missing Diagnosis, 3rd Edition.* Birmingham, AL: Missing Diagnosis, 1986.

Winter, Ruth. *A Consumer's Dictionary to Food Additives, 3rd Edition.* New York: Crown Publishers, 1987.

Wittenberg, Margaret M. *Experiencing Quality, A Shopper's Guide To Whole Foods.* Austin, TX: Whole Foods, 1987.

Wright, Jonathan V. *Dr. Wright's Book of Nutritional Therapy.* Emmaus, PN: Rodale Press, 1979.

General Index

Recipe Index

Index